"Take seven deep breaths... Al[...] captivating aromatic web—integr[...] [...] contained within holy texts as a means of exploring man's relationship with himself, with healing, with the divine, and with the wider world. It emphasizes scent as the cornerstone of integration of self, offering spiritual insights with a rare perspicacity."

—*Rhiannon Lewis, Editor of the*
International Journal of Clinical Aromatherapy

"Seven Scents distills the neuroscience and symbolism of fragrant plants to enrich our insight into a sense which, though trivialized by modern culture, unites the biological and spiritual. Professor Abram explores scented plant references in biblical and Hindu literature to reveal the wealth of meaning inherent in their stories. The sacred and therapeutic aspects of these narratives are sensitively compounded to awaken the reader's 'aromatic imagination'—and to tap the deepest roots of aromatherapy."

—*Gabriel Mojay Lic.Ac., CertEd, FIFPA, The Institute of*
Traditional Herbal Medicine & Aromatherapy (ITHMA)

"This presentation of seven scents in seven biographical case histories of religious figures that lived close to deity examines the integrative functioning of fragrance. Situated in a culturally determined context, scent is used as a pathway to spiritual transcendence. Abram offers a valuable observation on the loss of primordial consciousness and the role of perfume in a sanitized modern society. I recommend this book for anyone interested in the interaction of scent and spirituality."

—*Carl A.P. Ruck, author of* The Road to Eleusis:
Unveiling the Secret of the Mysteries

of related interest

FRAGRANCE AND WELLBEING

PLANT AROMATICS AND THEIR INFLUENCE ON THE PSYCHE
Jennifer Peace Rhind
ISBN 978 1 84819 090 0
eISBN 978 0 85701 073 5

AROMATHERAPEUTIC BLENDING

ESSENTIAL OILS IN SYNERGY
Jennifer Peace Rhind
ISBN 978 1 84819 227 0
eISBN 978 0 85701 174 9

THE SPIRIT IN AROMATHERAPY

WORKING WITH INTUITION
Gill Farrer-Halls
ISBN 978 1 84819 209 6
eISBN 978 0 85701 159 6

AROMATICA

A CLINICAL GUIDE TO ESSENTIAL OIL THERAPEUTICS.
VOLUME 1: PRINCIPLES AND PROFILES
Peter Holmes LAc, MH
ISBN 978 1 84819 303 1
eISBN 978 0 85701 257 9

SEVEN SCENTS

HEALING AND THE AROMATIC IMAGINATION

Dorothy P. Abram

Illustrations by Laura Mernoff

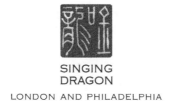

SINGING
DRAGON

LONDON AND PHILADELPHIA

First published in 2017
by Singing Dragon
an imprint of Jessica Kingsley Publishers
73 Collier Street
London N1 9BE, UK
and
400 Market Street, Suite 400
Philadelphia, PA 19106, USA

www.singingdragon.com

Library of Congress Cataloging in Publication Data
Title: Seven scents : healing and the aromatic imagination / Dorothy P. Abram ; illustrations by Laura Mernoff.
Description: London ; Philadelphia : Singing Dragon, 2017. | Includes bibliographical references.
Identifiers: LCCN 2016056182 | ISBN 9781848193499 (alk. paper)
Subjects: LCSH: Aromatic plants. | Aromatherapy. | Aromatherapy--History.
Classification: LCC SB301 .A27 2017 | DDC 635.9/68--dc23 LC record available at https://lccn.loc.gov/2016056182

British Library Cataloguing in Publication Data
A CIP catalogue record for this book is available from the British Library

ISBN 978 1 84819 349 9
eISBN 978 0 85701 307 1

Printed and bound in Great Britain

To
Daniel and Arianna
with love

*The fabled musk deer searches the world over for
the source of the scent which comes from itself.*

RAMAKRISHNA

CONTENTS

ACKNOWLEDGMENTS

I have had the pleasure of sharing this aromatic journey with friends and acquaintances who helped me along this route and deserve my sincere acknowledgement and gratitude.

First, my thanks to David Newman, chair of the Social Sciences department at Johnson & Wales University, who first recognized the possibility and promise of a book and encouraged me to pursue this pathway. Thanks to Johnson & Wales University that awarded me the Faculty Research Fellowship that afforded me the necessary time to devote to this project. Thanks to Christopher Westgate, too, for his feedback.

My gratitude to the editors at Singing Dragon Publishers, Jessica Kingsley and Sarah Hamlin, for their early and consistent support. Thanks, too, to my Long Table Writers Group: Kate Lohman, David Fox, Jim English, Jim Stahl, Barry Marshall, Susan Shepard, and Nick Boke for feedback and ongoing encouragement.

Thanks to Hananya Goodman, an extraordinary research librarian, who not only located relevant resources but also shared the delight of discovery with fragrance and scent with me. I also send my appreciation to Rhiannon Lewis and Gabriel Mojay, editors of the *International Journal of*

Clinical Aromatherapy, who published versions of two of the chapters and encouraged this perspective I employ. I also appreciate Laura Mernoff's talent and her willingness to provide illustrations for this book.

I am indebted to Swami Yogatmananda of the Vedanta Society of Providence and Sister Shuddhatmamata who were generous in my consultations with them and patient as I played with possibilities of interpretations. My appreciation also goes to Valerie Cooksley of the Institute of Integrative Aromatherapy who taught me clinical aromatherapy.

My thanks to friends and relatives who endured early drafts of this work: Tony Pappas, Izo Abram, Pat Overdeep, Suchismita Basu, Sravani Bhattacharjee, Abhijit Sarkar, Abhishek and Shuchi Goswami, and the Acharya family of Bhutan and Nepal who currently live in Columbus, Ohio.

And I give the greatest thanks to my husband Sam for his ardent and enthusiastic encouragement and support of this work.

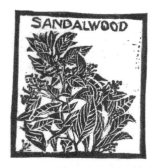
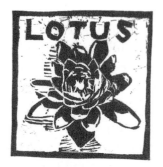
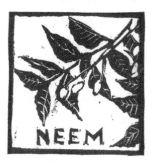
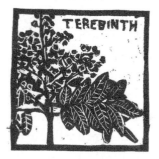
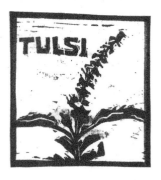
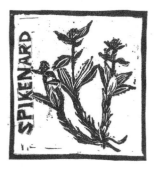
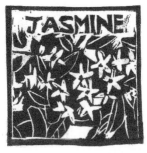

INTRODUCTION

The interrelationship between humans and plants has been a core aspect of their evolutions, each depending on the other for their growth, reproduction, survival, and flourishing.[1] More than simply providing food for humans, plants have also satisfied the human desire for transcendence—that is, to experience worlds of healing, wonder, and divinity beyond the limitations and restrictions of ordinary perception. At the same time, the senses, especially scent, which is the theme of this book, have also been used as a springboard into that unseen realm. Sacred texts, across traditions, repeatedly cite scent and aromatic plants as vehicles for accessing divine consciousness.[2] The interconnectedness of human and plant to achieve and provide conditions of healing and higher states of awareness in both biblical and Hindu traditions is the focus of this work.

I have chosen to examine seven aromatic plants—flowers and trees—and the lives of people whose stories intersect at crucial moments in their life journeys with these plants.

---

1   See Harari 2015; Pollan 2001; Stoddard 1991.
2   The research on this topic is wide-ranging: Bradley 2015; Classen, Howes and Synnott 1994; Green 2011; Harvey 2006; Manniche and Forman 1999; McHugh 2012; Reinarz 2014; Wasson, Ruck, and Hofmann 1978.

Healing is the goal of these narratives, whether physical, psychological, or spiritual. Healing in one of these dimensions recurrently heals the imbalances of the others. Oftentimes experienced within a setting of divine communication, the healing properties of the plants are made especially potent by the narrative that is attached to the curative context. The seven plants are: sandalwood (*Santalum album*), lotus (*Nymphaea caerulea*), neem (*Azadirachta indica*), terebinth (*Pistacia terebinthus*), tulsi (*Ocimum sanctum*), spikenard (*Nardostachys jatamansi*), and jasmine (*Jasminum officinale*).

BACKGROUND

I entered this study through an interest in ancient Greek mythology. I had the good fortune to study Greek language and literature as an undergraduate student with an inspirational professor who was dedicated to the relevance of ancient mythology to our lives today. He communicated his love of antiquity in a way that changed my life and some other lives of those studying with him. Professor Carl Ruck, with Albert Hoffman and R. Gordon Wasson, unraveled the significance of the ancient Greek mystery religion at the site of Eleusis in Greece.[3] Specifically, Carl and his colleagues examined the ritual use of ergot, a natural entheogen (hallucinogen) that inspired religious visions and spiritual realization in antiquity.

Years later, my work and studies led to my involvement with the Nepalese-Bhutanese refugee community who have recently resettled since 2007 in Providence, RI, USA, where I live. They brought with them rich cultural and religious traditions that used plants as central motifs in their worship

---

3   Wasson, Ruck, and Hofmann 1978. On entheogens, see Hoffman (2016); Ruck *et al.* (1976).

and in their everyday lives. Importantly, they generously and graciously welcomed me into their homes and patiently taught me their ways and traditions.[4] What had been previously an academic study of ritual and plants became for me, with these people, a living and vital performance of religious belief. Certainly, the stories from Hinduism included in this study owe much of their inspiration and knowledge to these beloved friends.

Making use of my advanced degrees in art and archaeology, in psychology, and in education, I returned to my early interest in ancient plant therapy in myth and ritual. It seemed to me that an appropriate route to further my knowledge of therapeutic and psychoactive plant use was to take an intensive course in aromatherapy that is employed in contemporary clinical settings. The therapeutic employment of aromatic plants through breath and other forms of ingestion are precisely the methods of healing that were used throughout the world in antiquity and in many contemporary world cultures. I discovered that it was only through experiencing diverse cultural methods that I could approach an understanding of therapeutic plant use in ancient and modern times. Indeed, through using knowledge of aromatic healing, I was able to decode and decipher ancient texts in ways that were previously inaccessible to scholarship. Looking at the plants and their effects through the lens of healing served to divulge themes and meanings, controversies and contradictions, and sentiments and significances that otherwise rested in shadows, undetected in traditional interpretations of these texts.

My writing on healing plants did not begin with intention or by design. Instead, I looked into various plants, images,

4   Abram 2015, forthcoming.

and personalities and these seven seemed fruitful. The seven chapters were written separately and independently of each other, as distinct studies on the healing capacities of each plant. After completing these seven separate essays, I recognized shared themes and overlapping narratives. Scent was vital to the experience of integration. Scent motivated on the physical level what was invoked in the mental, emotional, and spiritual domains.

Why scent? Why should scent be the sole sense that accomplishes this integration of self? Why not sight, or sound, or touch, or taste?

On one level, it might be said that attention to the senses—any and all—retrieves a neglect that has been fundamental to the history of Western philosophy. Scent, however, holds a special designation, that is, smell has been identified scientifically and historically as *the* sense that had to be repressed in order to achieve our human existence and identity. Relinquishing a four-footed method of locomotion, the human upright gait necessitated the renunciation of smell in favor of sight.

Thus, the repression of smell as a primary sensory mode is fundamental to our humanity. Scent, hereby, offers the possibility to retrieve that primordial experience at the borderline of memory and consciousness. Smell holds the capacity to revisit that loss. In this way, the healing knowledge brought about through scent serves to unite disparate identities—as animal and human—into a paradoxical unity. It asserts our animal origins while also affirming and enhancing our human identity. Opposites brought into union is the definition of *paradox* that is a focus of this book.

The unity that is implicit in the act of healing existential losses brings together the plant, its scent, its potency and mental effects with the individual experience in a cultural setting. Thereby, the union of mind, body, spirit, and community through the experience of scent is the ultimate expression of existential healing. This book is my journey through the magic, miracles, and mythologies of aromatic plants. My hope is that the reader becomes inspired to reintegrate scent into one's life to experience the vitality it offers. Before entering the study of the seven scents, it is important that I first examine the societal bias that frames and informs contemporary involvements with studies of scent.

RECLAIMING SCENT

Sociologist Georg Simmel made the claim that "The social question is not only an ethical one, but also a question of smell," and this is where our study begins.[5] When Freud traced the origin of the discontents of civilization, he located our existential dissatisfaction in an original separation from smell:

> The diminution of the olfactory stimuli seems itself to be a consequence of man's rising himself from the ground, of his assumption of an upright gait... From that point the chain of events would have proceeded through the devaluation of olfactory stimuli to the time when visual stimuli were paramount...and so to the threshold of human civilization.[6]

But don't blame Freud.

Ever since Freud located the origin of human discontent in repression of the olfactory sense, scholars have continued

---

5   Georg Simmel, quoted in Frisby and Featherstone 1997, p.118.
6   Freud 2010, p.78.

to neglect smell as a rich domain of inquiry in favor of the visual domain.

> Academic studies of smell have tended to suffer from the same cultural disadvantages as smell itself. While the high status of sight in the West makes it possible for studies of vision and visuality, even when they are critical, to be taken seriously, any attempt to examine smell runs the risk of being brushed off as frivolous and irrelevant.[7]

Freud followed Darwin's low estimation of the role of smell in human evolution. Both scholars echo Western philosophy—from Plato and Aristotle to Descartes, Kant, Schopenhauer, Hegel, and Simmel—in its rejection of the senses as legitimate and reliable sources of knowledge. Freud further extended his claim (that the repression of smell is the basis for civilization) to all strong scents as they are reminiscent, according to this psychoanalyst, of menses and excrement.[8] "It is an animal whose dominant sense is that of smell..." wrote Freud.[9] Thus, in rejecting smell, humans make their claim to being "civilized beings." But, at what cost? What is the price, both spiritual and psychological, that we pay for repressing a fundamental part of our senses and psyches and maintaining that repression?

Smell is the "fallen angel of the senses" wrote Helen Keller on this neglect of attention to scent in contemporary awareness.[10] Ignoring smell as a legitimate arena of inquiry deprives us of locating other possibilities of consciousness, sources of knowledge, and potentials for living. While vision maintains its elevated cultural status, in contrast to the

....

7   Classen *et al.* 1994, p.5.
8   Freud 2010, p.88.
9   Freud 2010, p.79, n.1.
10 Keller 2010, p.24, first published 1908.

rejection of scent, the opposition between the two senses perpetuates and reinforces long-standing dualities that have haunted Western philosophy. Oppositions such as culture versus nature, mind versus body, and those dualities of race, class, and gender act as a social hierarchy that reinforces inequities and stereotypes:

> Smell is consequently regarded as an essential ingredient in the emergence of larger dichotomies between peoples, such as that between Western and non-Western, colonizer and colonized, exploiter and exploited.[11]

Such categories are not natural, but socially constructed ethnocentric hierarchies that separate people from each other. Smell is used as a powerful means of stereotyping in this way.

As scent has been dismissed as a topic without interest to the majority of academics, the study of psychoactive and aromatic plants for healing purposes, accordingly, has been relegated to the field of aromatherapy. While aromatherapy has maintained old and ancient systems of healing, its use of the strong scents of aromatic plants necessarily has condemned it to an inferior status in the medical establishment characterized by sanitation, scent-neutrality, bourgeois aesthetics, and male-dominated medicine.[12] Ignoring fragrant therapeutic plants as sources of knowledge has thrown the field of aromatic healing into the hedonic sphere of the marketplace where aromatherapies flourish in commercial products from candles and perfumes to chocolates[13] and even sandwiches.[14]

11 Reinarz 2014, p.21; see also Classen, *et al.* 1994; Fiore 2015; Papenburg and Zarzycka 2013.
12 Corbin 1986; McClintock 1995; Sobchack 2013.
13 Marks 2013.
14 D'Angelo Restaurants advertisements 2016.

In each of these seven following chapters that span biblical and Hindu cultures, discontent, as Freud names the malaise of society, or what we might name "disability," is expressed as a ruptured consciousness and divided mind. It is cognitive dissonance (to use a contemporary psychological label) that undermines the integrity of the individual through divorcing thought and meaning from intention and action. Scent is used in specific narrative contexts to rectify this disruption, thereby reuniting the divisions of the self through embodied consciousness. Scent in the context of cultural significance bestows the individual with the capacity to heal divisions within the psyche and act toward human wholeness. That is the action of culturally situated psychoactive aromatic plants.

THE SOCIOLOGY OF SCENT

Even though each person enters this study with varied backgrounds, diverse engagements, and personal interactions with scent, it is important to consider the larger sociological context that frames these involvements. We live in a consumer capitalist economy that structures the identities and behaviors of its participants according to its own objectives and values, even as we are unconscious of its workings. In this environment, we experience scent as a commodity to be purchased. Furthermore, through this process, its participants assume the values necessary to fulfill its goals by experiencing scent through the lens of advertising, as Walter Benjamin notes: the "dream consciousness of the collective awakes in advertising."[15]

....
15 Quoted in Stamelman 2006, p.22.

The chapters that follow consider alternative models of engagement with fragrant plants. The identities developed through the cultural engagement of scent and psychoactive plants offer us insight into other ways of being than the consumer capitalist marketplace offers. How we experience scents, aromas, and smells reveals the biases of our society. Advertisements are coded means of communicating the marketplace's hidden ideological messages. It is important, then, to first explore the sociological setting of the current marketplace of scents and perfumes. Thereby, I want to clear the slate for an appreciation and celebration of alternative ways of being that studying psychoactive and therapeutic aromatic plants will open for us.

In the United States and in the West in general, we live in an antiseptic—a scentless—society. "Good sense is no scent" proclaims the signage of the movement to forbid the use of scents in public spaces. With growing commodification, societies increasingly deodorize, sanitize, and become aseptic. Personal habits and social mores follow. Scents naturally emitted from environments are replaced with heightened synthetic replicas to create simulated 'scentless' atmospheres and surroundings. I use the word *scentless* as a term to refer to society's ambivalence about smell. While fragrances have become a huge market, those smells replicate the dominant values of the society. Certain aromas are considered neutral or scentless though they actually have a distinct scent. Consider, in this way, the pine scent strip that is marketed for cars to be refreshed, or the recent fashion with perfumes that are "hygienic" or smell of "water."[16]

---

16 Ellena 2016, p.9.

Not all places and peoples in society, however, participate equally in this social ideology of scentlessness. Concurrently, poor or ethnic peoples and neighborhoods are considered "smelly" and socially segregated. The political use of smell as a social signifier of "otherness" through racial, ethnic, class, and gender oppression oftentimes inhibits an open discussion of smells because of the political sensitivity of the topic.[17] In the general population, the diminishing capacity to smell and perceive natural aromas—a condition called anosmia—is one profound consequence of this shift of sensibilities and aesthetics to scentlessness.

At the same time, scent is used to obscure smells that evoke and symbolize unwanted realities. The process of distancing the reality of waste, loss, deterioration, dying, and death, and its associated decay and stench, is the task of perfumes, a 40 billion dollar industry. Artificial scents and perfumes are created to "mask...unhappiness, depression, aging, illness, and death."[18] Accordingly, perfume advertising makes many promises: to awaken one's desire, passion, and purpose, to bestow happiness and sexual attraction, and to make one into one's own unattainable fantasies through the simple purchase of a perfume. The inevitable disappointment of that desire creates and fuels a cyclical purchasing process of dissatisfaction followed by the promise of the subsequent purchase to ease unhappiness. Thus, by identifying the values created by the advertising industry to promote aromatic scents, we are given a view of the inverted and repressed values of a consumer-capitalist society.

With its own symbols, images, and insights, the study of scent will reveal the repressed issues of a scentless society that not only neglects olfaction as a legitimate field of study, but is

17 Ackerman 1990, p.41.
18 Stamelman 2006, p.21.

also scent deprived. Perfume advertising is a central example of this notion of aroma playing the role of the "return of the repressed." Freud acknowledged that the repression of smell in the development of civilization had ongoing psychological and social implications. In his essays on *Moses and Monotheism* he explained that "what is forgotten is not extinguished, but only 'repressed'; its memory-traces are present in all their freshness, but isolated...they are unconscious."[19] Yet, at the same time, such repressed memories are constantly "re-emerging"[20] as "indications of a return of the repressed."[21] Modern advertising is a vehicle for articulating repressed emotional issues and concerns.

In a consumer-capitalist market culture, people are trained to seek answers to the pains of the heart and mind through what has been called "retail therapy": shopping. Note perfume company Bond No. 9's recent offer of a scent called *Madison Avenue*. It is advertised as "the world's first shopping fragrance."[22] Whereas other cultures, as will be shown, possess different models of responding to inherent contradictions that exist between individual experience and cultural norms, the advanced capitalist nations have chosen the context of the marketplace for healing.[23] Because the core issues are problems of the internal world, the capitalist promise of cure through externally purchasing more and newer "stuff"—and the latest expensive perfumes, for example—only perpetuates and exacerbates the divisions within. The suffering caused by the divided self has become a crisis of epidemic proportions.[24]

---

19 Freud 1939.
20 Rabain 2005.
21 Freud 1915.
22 *New York Times*, June 6, 2016, *NYT Beauty Magazine*.
23 Robbins 2005.
24 Sarno 2007.

PICKING UP THE SCENT:
SEARCHING FOR A SELF

The marketplace both creates and mirrors changing sensibilities and psychologies of the consumer. Scentlessness becomes a way of being. Perfume scholar Barbara Herman writes of the development of the "office scent" since the 1990s in perfumes: "an office scent's raison d'etre is to avoid being offensive. It plays well with others. By definition, it is institutional and conformist."[25] Herman cites Calvin Klein's best-selling 1994 unisex perfume *CK One* as a prime example of this notion of what I call a *scentless perfume* that "prolongs the feelings of being washed and clean." It is the scent of fresh "laundry."[26] Playing on this theme of scentless antisepsis, perfumer Moschino bottles his eau de toilette, called *Fresh Couture*, in a miniature glass Windex cleaning flacon.

It may not be a surprise then that Calvin Klein's next perfume was named *ck be*—with a scent designed to express "you." Hereby, the former perfume that was intended to comply with the scentless anonymity of society (*CK One*) is followed by a compensatory emphasis on individuality (*ck be*). *ck be* intends to bestow its wearer with a presence and a *being*. Klein astutely identified a contemporary existential challenge to reconcile "opposing forces." His advertisements for *ck be* spell out this struggle with duality. "be good. be bad. just be." urges one ad. "be hot. be cool. just be." says another. Whereas this study identifies the balance of oppositions as a spiritual and psychological goal, Klein's perfumes formulate that balance in a commercial product.

....

25 Herman 2013, p.5.
26 Burr 2007, pp.214, 250.

Promising to fulfill the desire for a self, an "I," amid the discontents of modern society, *ck be* is the perfect scent for today's "narcissistic person."[27] As with other scentless perfumes, *ck be* attempts to fulfill an existential need. "The individual atmosphere revealing the uniqueness of I must be allowed to break through" writes historian Alain Corbin of a similar consciousness in the 18th century.[28] Hereby, perfumes promise—but cannot deliver—material fulfillment of a non-material need.

Calvin Klein has again—a skill he has been celebrated for—"caught the mood of the moment."[29]

Or has he? *ck be* "tanked in the US market."[30] Was it the scent? Or, was it the message? Was there an inherent dissonance between the two that echoed a deeper division within?

Rather than containing the rich redolent scents of resinous and animalic base notes, these scentless perfumes are lighter and cleaner, creating cognitive and olfactory dissonance. The message does not match the scent, but, instead, corresponds to the scentless mentality of the marketplace. Transferring an emotional need into a purchasable commodity, perfume creates an endless cycle of buying motivated by dissatisfaction. The product claims to satisfy that dissatisfaction, but ultimately it cannot fulfill its promise. Such commodities do not—and cannot—supply the missing "I," but serve to exacerbate emotional divisions in their promise to do so.

The stories of scent in this collection also address the issue of a fundamental existential need, but in a manner that is

27 Fourquet-Courbet and Courbet 2007; Courbet and Fourquet-Courbet 2003; Grasse 2007.

28 Corbin 1986, pp.168, 177.

29 Dove 2014, p.233.

30 Burr 2007, p.158.

more substantive and satisfying. That need is treated with aromatic plant substances to heal a perceived absence within. The stories tell of an involvement that is so profound that it is oftentimes said to be an experience of the divine in the mortal realm. The outcome is an expansion of the self that creates a state of selflessness—a paradoxical unity of opposites that results in an expanded awareness of relationship and responsibility.

THE AROMATIC IMAGINATION

Individual experience of scent is personal and subjective. "Nothing" notes Diane Ackerman, "is more memorable than a smell. One scent can be unexpected, momentary, and fleeting, yet conjure up a childhood summer beside a lake in the mountains."[31] At the same time, scent is "culturally determined and collectively enacted."[32] The aromatic symbol-system, as scent itself, is culturally situated.

> The image system is part of the worldview of a culture; it taps into, and at the same time fashions and revises, the belief system and the repertoire of images which a culture stores and keeps ready for immediate use. The social strategies, the forms of perception, and the symbolic systems associated with the sense of smell participate in the formation from age to age of a scented imagination in which the real and sensory experience of [scent] is inextricably linked to the public's general awareness of what is real and sensory in the world.[33]

....

31 Ackerman 1990.
32 Stamelman 2006, p.21.
33 Stamelman 2006, p.22.

As do other symbol systems,[34] these aromatic stories reveal precise narrative codes specific to their own symbolic meanings.[35] This realization rests at the core of the aromatic imagination. Located within culture, scent seeks to redress inconsistencies of cultural experience—to release the repressed contents of the psyche. This aromatic imagination is expressed through its mending of emotional, psychological, and spiritual ruptures in social contexts. The healing of divisions, which is experienced through smell, is conveyed through narrative themes of unification of opposites in paradoxical relationship.

Each of the chapters that follow conveys this theme of paradoxical consciousness achieved through aromatic plants. The activation and efficacy of the aromatic imagination does not occur in isolation. It is part of a multidimensional complex of necessary elements to provide healing. The sense of smell works in conjunction with the psychoactive potencies of plants to create specific psychological states of consciousness. In addition, the narrative is supplied by the cultural context in interaction with the individual, and provides the basis for creating meaning. Each feature—mind, plant, person, story, context, and culture—is a necessary part of the larger construction of salience. Smell serves to secure the powerful experience of embodiment, bringing the outside world within. It is an inherently paradoxical arrangement; the outside (an aromatic plant) is brought within one's subjective realm of bodily perception and experience through its scent while simultaneously maintaining its objective status as an independent source of stimulation. Healing comes about through the integration and complementarity of these

34 Gardner 2011; Goodman 1976, 1978; Langer 1996.
35 Gilbert 2014.

elements, working in paradoxical conjunction, to create a whole. Hereby, we see that the mental effects of the aromatic plants replicate the narrative model of healing. The plant and the healing story overlap to create an intense coherence of meaning.

The question arises how we might engage healing narratives in society today. As traditional models are waning, and commercial capitalism depletes meaning, individuals are left on their own to find or to create their own pathways. In addition, the real power of story is experienced in community. What possibilities exist in contemporary times to retrieve these experiences as vital and salient? That is the question that each of us confronts even as we are left on our own, without shared mythic stories of meaning. This book invites us to look backwards to ancient times and sideways to other cultures to discover potential models of healing for our lives. Each story confronts its challenges differently, yet all were selected because of this common experience of the power of scent to create cognitive and spiritual unity.

Of course, reading about scent and scents is not the same as experiencing them first-hand (or, so to speak, by first-sniff). Certainly any scents that you acquire as companion to this study (sources listed in the Appendix) are not identical to those written about here, differing according to historical moment, provenance, harvest, and culture. Still, the attempt to accompany this study with actual scent is worth the effort and experience. My suggestion is to smell an absolute or essential oil version of the specific scents as you read the associated chapter. It will contribute a vital, dynamic, and irreplaceable experience of the story and it will ignite your own aromatic imagination.

BIBLIOGRAPHY

Abram, D. (2015) "The Cooking Lesson: Identity and Spirituality in the Lives of Hindu Refugees in America." In T. Cassidy and F. Pasche Guignard (eds) *What's Cooking, Mom? Narratives about Food and Identity*. Toronto: Demeter Press.

Abram, D. (forthcoming) "Symbol and Sel-Roti: The Taste of Return in Women's Nepali-Bhutanese-Hindu Refugees' Identity and Ritual Performance." In T. Cassidy and F. Pasche Guignard (eds) *Moving Meals and Migrant Mothers*. Toronto: University of Toronto Press.

Ackerman, D. (1990) *A Natural History of the Senses*. New York: Random House.

Bradley, M. (ed.) (2015) *Smell and the Ancient Senses*. New York: Routledge.

Burr, C. (2007) *The Perfect Scent: A Year inside the Perfume Industry in Paris and New York*. New York: Henry Holt and Company.

Classen, C., Howes, D., and Synnott. A. (1994) *Aroma: The Cultural History of Smell*. London and New York: Routledge.

Corbin, A. (1986) *The Foul and the Fragrant and the French Social Imagination*. Cambridge, MA: Harvard University Press.

Courbet, D. and Fourquet-Courbet, M-P. (2003) "Publicité, marketing, et parfums: approche psychosociale d'une double illusion." *Communication et Langages 136*, 43–57.

Dove, R. (2014) *The Essence of Perfume*. London: Black Dog Publishing.

Ellena, J-C. (2016) *Perfume: The Alchemy of Scent*. New York: Arcade Publishing.

Fiore, E. (2015) "Material Reconfiguration(s) of Racegender Entanglements: The Case of Rome's Banglatown." Research Master in Gender and Ethnicity, Institute for Cultural Inquiry, Utrecht University.

Fourquet-Courbet, M-P. and Courbet, D. (2007) "Perfume Advertising and Marketing: Evolution and New Trends." In M. Grasse (ed.) *Perfume, a Global History: From the Origins to Today*. Paris: Smogy Art Publisher, pp.255–257.

Freud, S. (1915) "Repression." In J. Strachey (ed.) *The Standard Edition of the Complete Psychological Works of Sigmund Freud*, pp.141–158.

Freud, S. (1939) "Moses and Monotheism: Three Essays." In J. Strachey (ed.) *The Standard Edition of the Complete Psychological Works of Sigmund Freud*, pp.1–137.

Freud, S. (2010) *Civilization and its Discontents*. New York and London: W.W. Norton. (Original work published 1930.)

Frisby, D. and Featherstone, M. (1997) *Simmel on Culture: Selected Writings*. London: Sage.

Gardner, H. (2011) *Frames of Mind: The Theory of Multiple Intelligences*. New York: Basic Books.

Gilbert, A. (2014) *What the Nose Knows: The Science of Scent in Everyday Life*. New York: Crown Publishers.

Goodman, N. (1976) *Languages of Art*. New York: Hackett Publishing.

Goodman, N. (1978) *Ways of Worldmaking*. New York: Hackett Publishing.

Grasse, M.C. (ed.) (2007) *Perfume, a Global History: From the Origins to Today*. Paris: Smogy Art Publishers.

Green, D.A. (2011) *The Aroma of Righteousness: Scent and Seduction in Rabbinic Life and Literature*. University Park, PA: The Pennsylvania State University Press.

Harari, Y.N. (2015) *Sapiens: A Brief History of Humankind*. New York: Harper.

Harvey, S.A. (2006) *Scenting Salvation: Ancient Christianity and the Olfactory Imagination*. Berkeley, CA: University of California Press.

Herman, B. (2013) *Scent and Subversion: Decoding a Century of Provocative Perfume*. Guilford, CN: Lyons Press.

Hoffman, M. (2016) "Entheogens (Psychedelic Drugs) and the Ancient Mystery Religions." In P. Wexler (ed.) *History of Toxicology and Environmental Health: Toxicology in Antiquity*, volume 2. Amsterdam: Elsevier Science Publishing, pp.126-135.

Keller, H. (2010) *The World I Live In*. (Original work published 1908.)

Langer, S. (1996) *Philosophy in a New Key*. Cambridge, MA: Harvard University Press.

Manniche, L. and Forman, W. (1999) *Sacred Luxuries: Fragrance, Aromatherapy, and Cosmetics in Ancient Egypt*. Ithaka, NY: Cornell University Press.

Marks, L.U. (2013) "Rethinking Multisensory Culture." In B. Papenburg and M. Zarzycka (eds) *Carnal Aesthetics: Transgressive Imagery and Feminist Politics*. London: I.B. Tauris, pp.144-157.

McClintock, A. (1995) *Imperial Leather: Race, Gender, and Sexuality in the Colonial Conquest*. New York: Routledge.

McHugh, J. (2012) *Sandalwood and Carrion Smell in Indian Religion and Culture*. New York: Oxford University Press.

Papenburg, B. and Zarzycka, M. (eds) (2013) *Carnal Aesthetics: Transgressive Imagery and Feminist Politics*. London: I.B. Tauris.

Pollan, M. (2001) *The Botany of Desire: A Plant's-Eye View of the World*. New York: Random House.

Rabain, J-F. (2005) "Return of the Repressed." In *International Dictionary of Psychoanalysis*. Encyclopedia.com. Accessed on 8 Aug 2016 at www. encylopedia.com.

Robbins, R. (2005) *Global Problems and the Culture of Capitalism*. Boston, MA: Pearson.

Reinarz, J. (2014) *Past Scents: Historical Perspectives on Smell*. Boston, MA: Pearson.

Ruck, C.A.P., Bigwood, J., Staples, D., Ott, J., and Wasson, G. (1976) "Entheogens." *Psychedelic Drugs 11*, 1-2, 145-146.

Sarno, J. (2007) *Divided Mind: The Epidemic of Mind Body Disorders*. New York: Harper Perennial.

Sobchack, V. (2013) "The Dream Olfactory: On Making Scents of Cinema." In B. Papenburg and M. Zarzycka (eds) *Carnal Aesthetics: Transgressive Imagery and Feminist Politics*. London: I.B. Tauris, pp.121-143.

Stamelman, R. (2006) *Perfume: Joy, Obsession, Scandal, Sin*. New York: Rizzoli International Publications.

Stoddard, D.M. (1991) *The Scented Ape: The Biology and Culture of Human Odour*. Cambridge: Cambridge University Press.

Wasson, R.G., Ruck, C., and Hofmann, A. (1978) *The Road to Eleusis: Unveiling the Secret of the Mysteries*. New York: Harcourt Brace Jovanovich.

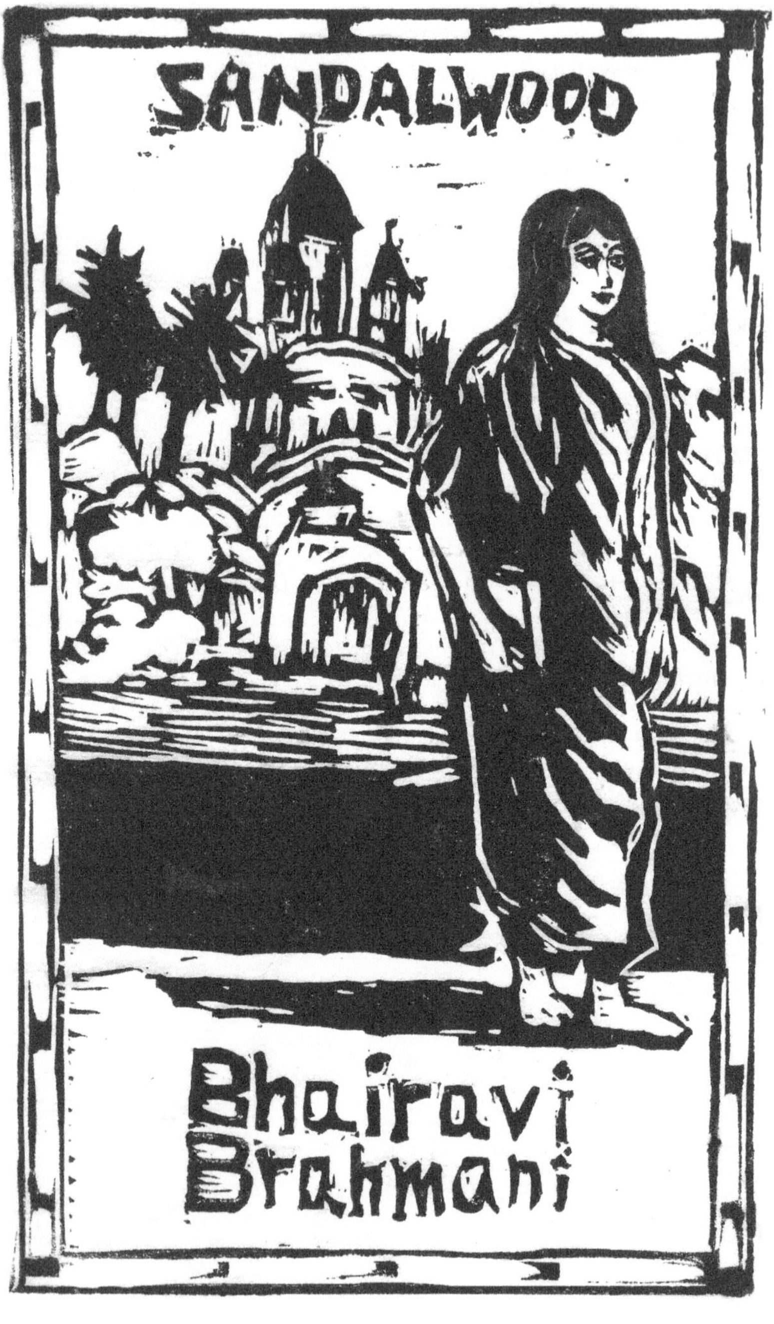
SANDALWOOD
Bhairavi
Brahmani

CHAPTER 1

BESMEARED WITH
SANDALWOOD

*Context, Culture, and Consciousness of Aromatic
Healing in the Life of a 19th-Century Hindu Saint*

INTRODUCTION

This chapter on sandalwood (*Santalum album*) presents a personal history of a 19th-century Hindu priest in which cognitive disunity is a mental illness that ultimately is healed through divine identification and the union of mortal and divine in a paradoxical identity. I focus on the priestess Bhairavi Brahmani's healing of the insanity of the 19th-century Hindu saint Ramakrishna through her use of *Santalum album* (sandalwood). Though numerous methods and approaches had been used previously by others in attempts to cure Ramakrishna, it was her particular approach and treatment that worked to heal this priest and to enable him to develop into his role as teacher, leader, and saint.

The chapter examines Bhairavi's healing methods. It also considers the potencies of sandalwood that were employed effectively for his disorder. In addition, the chapter emphasizes the necessity of understanding the cultural context in which diagnosis and treatment are accomplished. Curative outcomes necessarily depend on cultural and personal narratives that provide the emotional, mental, and spiritual significance and efficacy of healing. For both Bhairavi and Ramakrishna, their engagement with the restorative effects of sandalwood proved to be a great creative cultural act that demonstrated their authority in their religious community. Bhairavi's treatment and cure of Ramakrishna with sandalwood assured her historical notice and survival as one of the great figures of aromatic healing. Thus, sandalwood is the means of Ramakrishna's cure from madness, but it is the narrative context in which the cure is offered whereby its healing effects are secured.

THE MADNESS OF RAMAKRISHNA

The year was 1861 and the place was at the shore of the Ganges River in India. A beautiful middle-aged woman with disheveled hair, dressed in ochre robes and carrying a book, arrived at the Dakshineswar Temple of the Hindu goddess Kali. Her title was Bhairavi Brahmani. She was looking for Ramakrishna, the priest of the temple, to treat his fever and delusions. Her prescribed treatment was to use sandalwood paste.

This historical vignette relates the story of Bhairavi Brahmani and it is almost all we know about this woman who transformed religious history. We don't know how she knew about Ramakrishna's disorder or if she was sent by someone else for this purpose. In fact, we wouldn't have known even these few facts about Bhairavi had it not been for her entry into the life of the 19th-century Bengali saint named Ramakrishna.

Considered strange by some and insane by others, Ramakrishna experienced visions and trances from a young age. These disruptions of consciousness became increasingly frequent as he became older. Ramakrishna's frustration over his inability to control his mental, physical, emotional, and spiritual disability led him to attempt suicide. When Ramakrishna's older brother Ramkumar died unexpectedly, Ramakrishna, as a Brahmin, was asked to replace him as the priest of the Hindu goddess Kali at her temple at Dakshineswar.

It was there that Ramakrishna first experienced an inexorable and unrelenting fever. A disciple describes Ramakrishna's suffering:

> Sometime before the Brahmani arrived, the Master had been suffering terribly from an intense burning sensation all over his body. Treatments of many sorts were administered but the cure was as far away as ever. We were told by the Master himself that the pain, starting with sunrise, went on increasing as the day advanced, till it became unbearable by midday, when he had to keep his body immersed in the water of the Ganga for two or three hours, with a wet towel placed on his head. He had to come out of the water even against his will, lest he should fall a prey to some other disease because of cold.[1]

Based on Ramakrishna's complaints of overwhelming heat and his symptoms, Bhairavi chose aromatherapy; that is, she decided to employ a paste of *Santalum album* (white sandalwood, in Sanskrit called *chandana*) to apply "for three days." As a paste, sandalwood's thermal conductive properties draw heat away from the body and, thereby, create the effect

---

1   Saradananda 1952, p.574.

and sensation of coolness. Simultaneously, it transfers its active ingredient through transdermal absorption.[2] Recent dermatological research has found that sandalwood activates chemical sensors on the surface of the skin that pick up the same chemicals as scent receptors to provide healing effects.[3] In Ayurvedic medicine, sandalwood is a cooling agent that is used in paste form and "applied to the foreheads of people suffering from fever."[4] Bhairavi's prescription was consistent with contemporary and current medical knowledge. Indeed, sandalwood is used popularly in a similar manner in India today where sandalwood soap is preferred for use in the summertime heat; in contrast, glycerin soap is chosen in the winter for its thermal properties as a heat-retaining agent.[5]

We might wonder how this application of a paste on the skin could be more effective than the chilly Himalayan waters of the Ganges in which Ramakrishna spent many hours and days to cool himself. Bhairavi's chosen regimen of sandalwood paste, however, was not the entire extent of her treatment program. She was a magnificent holistic healer who understood the multidimensionality of illness and, accordingly, the multifaceted treatment that was necessary. Her healing approach involved spiritual transformation whereby "the 'bonds' of men are turned into 'releasers.' The very poison that kills is transmuted into the elixir of life."[6] Bhairavi presents us with a compelling narrative of meaning and purpose to restructure Ramakrishna's perception of his "disease."

....

2   Hongratanaworakit 2004; Hongratanaworakit, Heuberger and Buchbauer 2004.
3   Busse 2014.
4   Kapoor 2001, p.26.
5   My thanks to Mita Basu for this information.
6   Nikhilananda in Gupta 1942, p.26.

SANDALWOOD: SIGNS AND SIGNATURES

The paste Bhairavi prepared is employed regularly in worship of Hindu deities. Ground wood mixed with water on a flat stone, the paste is used to mark the flowers offered to the deities and to anoint the brows of idols, acknowledging and signaling their divinity. This fragrant designation of divinity is crucial to understanding the cultural symbolism and religious use of sandalwood. Traditionally, sandalwood indicates the auspiciousness of the sacred and that auspiciousness is signaled by a pleasing scent. All the gods, except for the formidable deity Kali who is marked with red sandalwood, are designated with the sign of white sandalwood. Sandalwood is a superlative medium that cannot be superseded by any other. The mystic poet Sri Jynaneshwar (1275-1296 CE) stated this with his famous question, "With what kind of perfume can you besmear the sandalwood tree?" In other words, nothing is greater than sandalwood.

For Meera (1498-c.1546), also called Mirabai, a female mystic of the 16th century, such ritual gestures were more than compulsory acts: "whenever she had a chance she would apply sandalwood at the forehead of the God's statue and prepare garlands for the offerings."[7] Clearly, these ritual actions were sources of great pleasure and earned Meera so much karmic merit that she, it was told, did not die, but simply merged into the consciousness of Krishna.[8]

Bhairavi used sandalwood and a floral garland, placed around Ramakrishna's neck, as the elements of his treatment. Swami Saradananda, a disciple of Ramakrishna, tells us that "the medicine for this so called 'disease' was also extraordinary,

7   Prabhune 2012.
8   Bly and Hirshfield 2004, p.81.

viz, to adorn the patient with sweet-smelling flowers and to smear his body with fragrant sandal-paste."[9]

Although we are not told the specific names of those "sweet-smelling flowers," other sources inform us that it was a garland like the ones put on the temple's idols every day; in addition to their own floral fragrance, these flowers also carried the scent of sandalwood. As we saw with the mystic Meera above, to make a ritual object appropriate for dedication to the gods, each flower of the garland must be touched with sandalwood. The sandalwood scent of Ramakrishna's garland thus derived from its ritual preparation, in addition to the fragrant flowers gathered from the garden. Through this means, Bhairavi enhanced the effects of her sandalwood paste with sandalwood inhalation. This modality would have been further amplified by the sandalwood incense smoke that filled and fragranced the sanctuary.

HEALING PROPERTIES OF SANDALWOOD

Sandalwood's medicinal properties are anti-inflammatory, hypotensive, and sedative, reducing stress, anxiety, and depression.[10] A hemiparasitic tree that is native to India and Indonesia, sandalwood achieves maturity at 60 years when its essential oil, contained in its heartwood, reaches its full potency. The heartwood contains up to 90 percent sesquiterpenoid sanatol alchohols, the active ingredient in treating mental dysfunctions and physical disorders of a divided mind and split consciousness.[11] In fact, researchers

....
9   Saradananda 1952, p.574.
10 Battaglia 2003; Bhowmik, Biswas, and Kumar 2011.
11 Misra and Dey 2013, p.11; Battaglia 2003; Bieri, Monastyrskaia, and Schilling 2004.

have identified its similar properties, potency, and application with the neuroleptic and anti-psychotic drug chlorpromazine.[12] Recent research distinguishes between sandalwood's multiple healing capacities. Hongratanaworakit and his colleagues delineate the dual integrative potencies of sandalwood to treat body and mind:

> While a-sanatol [sandalwood's active ingredient] caused significant physiological changes which are interpreted in terms of relaxing/sedative effect, sandalwood oil provoked physiological deactivation but behavioral activation. These findings are likely to represent an uncoupling of physiological and behavioral arousal processes by sandalwood oil.[13]

Historical and aromatherapeutic inquiries, like this study of sandalwood and Hindu mysticism, offer us complementary narratives with scientific research to provide a fuller and more complex tale of healing.

With testimony about Ramakrishna's medical treatment for his fever just prior to Bhairavi's arrival, we witness what Bhairavi offered in contrast with traditional medical treatment that focused on symptoms without narrative meaning.

> None...it is superfluous to say, could suppress laughter at the Brahmani's "diagnosis of the disease," let alone the treatment suggested. They thought within themselves, "How preposterous it is for her to say it is not a disease, when it could not at all be alleviated even by taking so much medicine and using so many oils like Madhyamanarayana,

---

12 Bagchi and Kar 2011; Heuberger, Hongratanaworakit, and Buchbauer 2006; Okugawa *et al.* 1995.
13 Hongratanaworakit *et al.* 2000, p.3.

Vishnu, and the like!" But no one could have any possible objection to the simple, innocuous and easily-arranged treatment prescribed by the Brahmani. Everyone was sure that the patient himself would give it up in a day or two, finding it of no use. The person of the Master was accordingly adorned with sandal-paste and garlands of flowers following Brahmani's prescription; and to the astonishment of all, the burning sensation of the Master's body completely disappeared in three days.[14]

Like sandalwood, the specific Ayurvedic oil mixtures mentioned here (Vishnu oil and Madhyama Narayana oil) are prescribed for nervous disease and hypertension.[15] However, Ayurvedic medicine alone was inadequate for Ramakrishna's healing transformation; he required an integrated, narrative, and spiritually derived treatment and relationship that Bhairavi offered. Sandalwood was her means and aromatherapy was her method. Recent research on the bio-chemical activity of sandalwood on the brain suggests that this plant works on the perception of pain in addition to its effect on the body's pain pathways.[16] With this insight, we identify the necessity of examining Ramakrishna's mental involvement with his cure, and Bhairavi's manipulation of perception as part of her healing process.

NARRATIVE IDENTITIES

Clearly, Ramakrishna's core dilemma was not nervousness or anxiety that sandalwood paste or smoke inhalation might

14 Saradananda 1952, p.574.
15 Dutt 2012; Kapoor 2001.
16 Sari *et al.* 2013.

treat nor was it simply the sensation of physical heat. Instead, Ramakrishna was undergoing a crisis of a divided self; that is, a denial, according to Bhairavi, of his true nature and real self. As a monk from a local center of the Ramakrishna Order in Providence, RI, USA recently explained to me, Ramakrishna's illness was a "physical expression of a psychic condition."[17] Bhairavi's therapy first contextualized Ramakrishna's illness within a framework of normality. She "listened to him attentively and said: 'My son, everyone in this world is mad. Some are mad for money, some for creature comforts, some for name and fame; and you are mad for God.'"[18] Insanity, Bhairavi explained, is the human condition.

Bhairavi then presented Ramakrishna with a compelling narrative of meaning and purpose to treat his mind as well as body. Using relevant passages from Hindu sacred scriptures as evidence, Bhairavi claimed that Ramkrishna had demonstrated identical symptoms with the great sages Sri Radharani and Sri Chaitanya that Hindu religious traditions recognized as divine incarnations.[19] She believed Ramakrishna was the contemporary manifestation of God on earth.

Bhairavi's conviction of Ramakrishna's divinity from the life stories of Sri Radharani and Sri Chaitanya was the narrative framework that made sense of his behavior beyond mental illness. She not only legitimized his symptoms through these analogies, but she also provided a larger context of meaning. Bhairavi "came to the conclusion that such things [Ramakrishna's extraordinary experiences] were not possible for an ordinary devotee, not even for a highly developed soul. Only an Incarnation of God was capable

----

17 Yogatmananda 2014.
18 Gupta 1942, p.18.
19 Gupta 1942, p.19.

of such spiritual manifestations."[20] According to Bhairavi, Ramakrishna's mental state was an example of *mahabhava*, the great mystical realization of divine consciousness.[21] Bhairavi was adamant and unwavering, arguing her belief even before a committee convened to determine the truth of her assertions.[22]

Mahabhava, a transcendent state of consciousness, was a rapturous experience of the highest realization. From this psychological perspective, Ramakrishna's suffering was the result of a divided mind in his denial and rejection of this identity that, as consequence, locked him into a feverish illness of imbalance. By providing him with an affirming and transcendent narrative of the significance of his madness, Bhairavi connected Ramakrishna to his existential meaning and purpose. Bhairavi reformulated his experience as a choice on a spectrum of reasonable and positive options, thereby bestowing him with agency and authority to function and work, and to become a great spiritual leader: "she recognized in him a power to transmit spirituality to others."[23]

Her choice of cooling Ramakrishna through application of sandalwood was not an arbitrary or random selection. It had a long literary tradition. For example, consider this verse from a 16th-century devotional poem: "How can I heal myself, O my companion? I may crush cool sandalpaste and apply it..."[24] Sandal paste is a regularly repeated metaphor in this bhakti tradition of devotional poetry. Within the concept of coolness, as opposed to heat, are the associated values of

....

20 Gupta 1942, p.18.
21 McDaniel 1989.
22 Saradananda 1952.
23 Gupta 1942, p.19.
24 Alston 2008, p.36.

divine versus human.[25] The divine is identified with coolness and fragrance (and other associated dualities), in opposition to the decay and stench of mortal life as it moves inevitably to death. Sandalwood, in color, scent, and effect (coolness), replicates the dimensions and sensibilities of divine identity. It is no surprise then that statues of Hindu gods are carved in fragrant sandalwood. "In that wood [sandal] lives our beloved," writes the mystic poet, "The wood that gives out the scent of sandalwood."[26]

RITUAL ACTS: PERFORMING IDENTITY

In addition, we must consider the religious significance of this healing act as ritual performance. As perfume scholar Jellinek explains, "aromas are experienced within the context of life situations,"[27] and the context within which Ramakrishna received his sandalwood paste treatment is particular to Hindu worship and ritual. Bhairavi's use of sandalwood scent was contextualized within a meaningful religious practice and performance. Her placement of a garland of flowers around Ramakrishna's neck replicates the duty that Ramakrishna performed each morning for the statues of the gods. He gathered flowers from the temple garden, touched them with sandalwood, encircled each statue with this floral dedication, and besmeared the idols with sandalwood, devotedly acknowledging the divinity of each god in the human world. Bhairavi, hereby, repeated this same gesture in treating Ramakrishna with the sandal paste and garland that she adorns him with, just as the Hindu saint Sri Chaitanya

---

25 McHugh 2012.
26 Esmail 2002, p.89.
27 Jellinek 1998, p.115.

had done during his own *mahabhava*. As performance of the highest spiritual level, Bhairavi enacted Ramakrishna's transformation: thus, instead of being the subject in the act of devotion to the gods, Ramakrishna was made into the object of devotion as God incarnate and, consequently, besmeared with sandalwood paste.

Ramakrishna's experience of healing through sandalwood paste application resonates meaningfully on many levels within his religious framework. To experience that coolness is to affirm experientially the religious values that Ramakrishna practiced, including the belief that divinity rests within the individual and the devotee's challenge in life is to realize this truth. Bhairavi's purposeful use of sandalwood brought that unity into fruition through authentic experience. Ramakrishna's disabling heat signaled his distance from his divine identity as a disability that afflicted him. Coolness, as a characteristic of divine identity, was the state of body and mind that Bhairavi had to effect through her treatment to heal Ramakrishna.

Indeed, we notice the role of sandalwood in this same spiritual formulation and interpretation in the lives of other Hindu saints. For example, Mirabei, a 16th-century female saint, used sandalwood to poetically convey her desire for unity with her god, Krishna, through the ritual of mixing sandalwood paste. When she writes, "You are the sandalwood, I am the water...," Mirabei uses the same metaphor of the ritual mixing of sandalwood paste to describe mystical unity. Clearly, the only consciousness that surpasses the coolness of sandalwood is mystical union, as another female mystic tells us about her desire to unite with Krishna, "The flowers and the sandalwood are in vain and without effect. They fail to cool my burning for him, and I dislike all than the dear son of Devaki [Krishna]."[28] This is the metaphorical and spiritual reality into which Bhairavi led Ramakrishna. In doing this, Ramakrishna claimed his true identity and his mental illness was transformed from disability to superlative ability. As tradition prescribed, Ramakrishna found his faith and his god: within himself. For three years, Ramakrishna studied with Bhairavi and then, once again, Bhairavi disappears from the historical record.

CULTURE AND CREATIVITY

Bhairavi employed sandalwood to address bodily concerns and used sacred history to provide narratives of meaning. A final challenge remained to situate Ramakrishna's experience within a cultural context to connect with his community. To witness Bhairavi's healing insight in this dimension, we must consider how creativity functions in the collective society in which they lived.

To ignore Bhairavi's therapy—and Ramakrishna's subsequent teaching—as anything less than a great creative accomplishment would be a serious oversight. Creativity is often defined by Western writers working within an individualistic society as a solitary activity resulting in a product that changes the status quo in which the artist produces.[29] However, through this definition, we neglect to understand the creative accomplishments of both Bhairavi and Ramakrishna. Creativity within a collectivist culture manifests according to the values of collectivism.[30] Thus, creativity is re-construction (rather than innovation) of traditional

....

28 Prabhune 2012, p.14.
29 Misra, Srivastava, and Misra 2006.
30 Bhawuk 2003; Hofstede 1980; Livermore 2009.

belief or practice toward continuing religious experience.[31] Rather than rejecting the values of their society, collectivist creators confirm its premises with a creative reworking of its expressions and experiences. We see this in Ramakrishna's account of the direction of his transformation: "Hitherto he had pursued his spiritual ideal according to the prompting of his own mind and heart. Now he accepted [Bhairavi] Brahmani as his guru and set foot on the traditional pathways."[32]

Bhairavi also used traditional medical methods, religious beliefs, and historical narrative (all involving sandalwood) to rework an understanding of Ramakrishna's madness through her intellect, intuition, compassion, connection, and creativity. According to Saradananda, as we've already seen, Bhairavi, from the start, recognized Ramakrishna's capacity to sustain the community and teach their collective about the unity of life. Hers was a sandalwood cooling method that connected humanity with the divine through the transformed consciousness of a Bengali saint.

CONCLUSION

In this examination of sandalwood, Bhairavi offered many lessons using sandalwood as the means, method, and model of spiritual enlightenment and aromatic healing. First, Bhairavi recognized the ultimate unity of mind, body, and spirit that was demonstrated through her use of sandalwood paste to treat Ramakrishna and cure his suffering on these multiple levels synchronously. Second, by recognizing and renaming Ramakrishna's assumed madness as manifestation of the great religious realization of the saints, Bhairavi offered

---

31 Bhawuk 2003.
32 Gupta 1942, p.20.

Ramakrishna a narrative affirmation and integration of his experience, thereby enabling Ramakrishna's authority and agency to teach the power of the unseen world in human life. Third, Bhairavi performed her treatment within a meaningful cultural context of connection and creativity through aromatic healing and spiritual insight. She prescribed sandalwood paste (that is applied daily to the images of the gods) for Ramakrishna, thereby reversing the roles of devotee and Divine, in performative demonstration of transformation and transcendence. A final lesson from this study is that culture runs deep and oftentimes its workings rest out of sight. As aromatherapists, we must delve into the systems of meaning that provide contexts for understanding people and plants, and that, at the same time, offer systems of meaning that enable healing.

BIBLIOGRAPHY

Alston, A. (2008) *The Devotional Poems of Mirabai*. Delhi: Motilal Banarsidass Publishers.

Bagchi, P. and Kar, A. (2011) "Ayur-informatics: establishing an in-silico-Ayurvedic medication and RNAi treatment for schizophrenia." *Journal of Bioscience and Technology 2*, 1, 205-212.

Basu, S. (July 13, 2014) Personal communication. Kolkata, India and Providence, RI, USA.

Battaglia, S. (2003) *The Complete Guide to Aromatherapy*. Brisbane, Australia: The International Centre of Holistic Aromatherapy.

Bhawuk, D. (2003) "Culture's influence on creativity: the case of Indian spirituality." *International Journal of Intercultural Relations 27*, 1-22.

Bhowmik, D., Biswas, D., and Kumar, K. (2011) "Recent aspect of ethnobotanical application and medicinal properties of traditional Indian herbs santalum album." *International Journal of Chemistry Research 1*, 2, 2-27.

Bieri, S., Monastyrskaia, K., and Schilling, B. (2004) "Olfactory receptor neuron profiling using sandalwood odorants." *Chemical Senses 29*, 483-487.

Bly, R. and Hirschfield, J. (2004) *Mirabai Ecstatic Poems*. Boston, MA: Beacon Press.

Bobde, P. (1995) *Garland of Divine Flowers: Selected Devotional Lyrics of Saint Jnanesvara*. Delhi: Motilal Banarsidass Publishers.

Busse, D. (2014) "A synthetic sandalwood odorant induces wound-healing processes in human keratinocytes via the olfactory receptor OR2AT4." *Society for Investigative Dermatology 134*, 2823-2832.

Dutt, U. (2012) *The Materia Medica of the Hindus*. Calcutta: Thacker, Spink & Co.

Esmail, A. (2002) *A Scent of Sandalwood: Indo-Ismaili Religious Lyrics*. London: Curzon Press.

Gupta, M. (1942) *The Gospel of Sri Ramakrishna*. New York: Ramakrishna-Vivekananda Center.

Heuberger, E., Hongratanaworakit, T., and Buchbauer, G. (2006) "East Indian Sandalwood and a-santalol odor increase physiological and self-rated arousal in humans." *Planta Medica 72*, 792-800.

Hofstede, G. (1980) *Culture's Consequence: Comparing Values, Behaviors, Institutions, and Organizations Across Nations*. Thousand Oaks, CA: Sage.

Hongratanaworakit, T. (2004) "Physiological effect in aromatherapy." *Songklanakarin Journal of Science and Technology 26*, 1.

Hongratanaworakit, T., Heuberger, E., and Buchbauer, G. (2004) "Evaluation of the effects of East Indian sandalwood oil and a-santalol on humans after transdermal absorption." *Planta Medica 70*, 1, 3-7.

Jellinek, J. (1998) "Odours and mental states." *International Journal of Aromatherapy 9*, 3, 115-120.

Kapoor, L. (2001) *Handbook of Ayurvedic Medicinal Plants*. London: CRC Press.

Kaufman, J. and Sternberg, R. (eds) (2006) *The International Handbook of Creativity*. Cambridge: Cambridge University Press.

Kumar, A., Arun, G., and Mohan Ram, H. (2012) "Sandalwood: history, uses, present status and the future." *Current Science 103*, 12.

Livermore, D. (2009) *Expand Your Borders*. Grand Rapids, MI: Baker Academic.

Markus, H. and Kitayama, S. (1991) "Culture and self: implications for cognition, emotion, and motivation." *Psychological Review 98*, 2, 224-253.

McDaniel, J. (1989) *The Madness of Saints: Ecstatic Religion in Bengal.* Chicago: University of Chicago Press.

McHugh, J. (2012) *Sandalwood and Carrion Smell in Indian Religion and Culture.* Oxford: Oxford University Press.

Misra, B. and Dey, S. (2013) "Biological activities of East Indian sandalwood tree, *santalum album." PeerJ PrePrints*, November 12.

Misra, G., Srivastava, K., and Misra, I. (2006) "Culture and Facets of Creativity: The Indian Experience." In J. Kaufman and R. Sternberg (eds) *The International Handbook of Creativity.* Cambridge: Cambridge University Press, pp.421–456.

Okugawa, H., Ueda, R., Matsumoto, K., Kawanishhi, K., and Kato, A. (1995) "Effect of a-sanatol and b-santalol from sandalwood on the central nervous system in mice." *Phytomedicine* 2, 2, 119–126.

Prabhune, S. (2012) *They Said It: Translations of the Poems of the Saint Poets.* Bloomington, IN: AuthorHouse.

Sanford, A. (2008) *Singing Krishna Sound Becomes Sight in Paramananda's Poetry.* New York: State University of New York Press.

Saradananda (1952) *Sri Ramakrishna The Great Master.* Chennai: Sri Ramakrishna Math.

Saradananda (2003) *Ramakrishna and His Divine Play.* St. Louis: Vedanta Society of Saint Louis.

Sari, K., Damayanti, A., Salikha, K., Yuliati, A., and Sjuhada, A. (2013) "Inhalation of sandalwood aromatherapy to divert pain perception." CISAK C4/O/39.

Snelling, A. (1993) *For Love of the Dark One: Songs of Mirabai.* Boston, MA: Shambala.

Spence, D. (1984) *Narrative Truth and Historical Truth: Meaning and Interpretation in Psychoanalysis.* New York: W.W. Norton.

Yogatmananda (August 15, 2014) Personal communication. Vedanta Society of Providence, RI, USA.

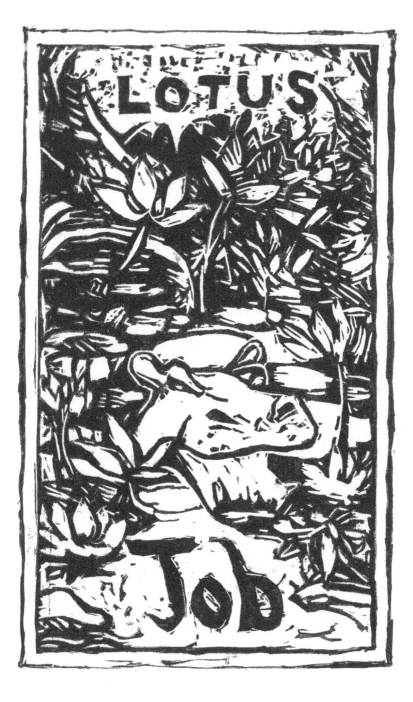

CHAPTER 2

SHAMANIC ASPECTS IN THE JOURNEY OF JOB

The Healer as Hero

INTRODUCTION

"There was a man in the land of Uz, whose name was Job..."[1] With this fairytale introduction, the book of Job begins.

The biblical figure of Job may seem an unexpected character by which to explore the theme of healing with aromatic plants. Indeed, this model came about quite serendipitously. Having been invited to present my work at an academic conference on shamanism and anthropology, I used the theme of the conference—shamanism—to explore the significance of the fragrant psychoactive lotus (water lily) that appears in the story of Job. The shaman is a religious specialist who journeys, typically traveling through ingestion (or through inhalation) of a psychoactive plant, into unseen realms of the spirit to rescue lost or abducted souls of the living. I wondered: could Job also be considered a shaman? If so, how could such

---

1   Job 1.1.

an unorthodox interpretation of this well-studied biblical book provide relevant and robust evidence? Moreover, how would such an unexpected interpretation contribute to this study of healing through scent today?

With these questions in mind, this chapter investigates the framework, form, and function of shamanic storytelling to analyze Job's role in the contest between God and the Adversary that is told in the biblical book of Job. I examine the identity of the shaman who, as spiritual healer, achieves a heightened state of consciousness to accomplish the goal of rescue and healing. The model of the shaman as archetypal healer has not been used previously to decipher the significance of this biblical book. However, the appearance of the sacred Egyptian lotus (or blue water lily) and the mythical hippopotamus in this text point in this direction of analysis. The aromatic scent and hypnotic effects of the lotus (lily) provide the model of psychological change that will prove to be among the shaman's tools of healing. Thus, Job's heroic challenge is essentially a psychological journey through darkness and his return into an integrated identity. I am not claiming that Job literally ingests the water lily or lotus; instead, the symbolic and metaphorical meaning of this scented flower shapes this story. The psychoactive effects define the narrative plot. We can recognize, then, that, in this context, scent signals descent and, through healing, scent indicates ascent as well.

THE JOURNEY AND THE SHAMAN

The story of Job was a primordial battle for truth and meaning—and Job was at the center of this existential struggle. Would Job prove the higher truth represented by his God? Or, would he demonstrate the depletion of meaning and purpose of human existence argued by the Adversary? This test of truth was accomplished through suffering. If Job could decipher its significance to prove the existence of a higher integrated consciousness, the battle would be decided in his favor. This, too, is the challenge that faces the healer today— that is, for patients to be able to interpret the meaning of suffering for their lives. This chapter cannot provide that answer, but, instead, focuses on the process of resolution of suffering through aromatic healing.

The shaman achieves his expertise by overcoming the very suffering, obstacles, and disabilities that define his skills as a healer.[2] The shaman's journey represents a psychological process of healing. Thus, we easily may see the ancient biblical figure of Job as a shaman—that is, as a person who suffers and, through his suffering, rescues and heals the world. Analysis of the book of Job provides additional evidence that confirms his identity as shamanic healer. This chapter examines that evidence to reveal the dimensions of knowledge and healing that this shamanic Job provides.

Scholars typically neglect to recognize or to examine Job's shamanic role, preferring instead to analyze him as a tortured hero of religious literature.[3] The text, however, reveals a specific shamanic identity. This identity integrates certain anomalies of the text in a manner that explains elements that are otherwise seen as disjointed or fragmented. By examining Job as a shaman, these components of the story are brought together to provide an integrated narration. I follow the evidence by examining five elements of shamanism: codes, magical plant, the journey, return, and three challenges.

The tale of Job begins with a contest and battle between God and the Adversary (Satan) over the true identity of

---

2   Eliade 1967; Fadiman 1997; Halifax 1982; Winkelman 2004.
3   Mitchell 1987; Pope 1973; Scheindlin 1998.

God's beloved worshiper Job. While God insists Job's piety is pure, the Adversary maintains that Job's faith is simply the outcome of the blessings that God has heaped upon his pious worshipper. Challenge Job with hardship, the Adversary claims, and his faith will disappear and he will curse God. Thus begins this battle for truth between unseen cosmic powers. The Adversary initiates the harassment of Job, destroying the lives of Job's children, wealth, power, property, and health. Job fights on behalf of God's reputation and human meaning, ultimately defeating the Adversary by refusing to curse God and by accepting the inscrutability of divine consciousness.

CODES AND CONTEXTS

Because of the narrative methods of the book of Job and the prehistoric origins of shamanic religious practice, the references to the shamanic experience are coded, symbolic, and allusive. For example, the book of Job is noted for its unusual use of language. Called *hapax legomena*, "things said once," words are used in this biblical book that are not seen elsewhere in the entire Bible.[4] One example is what is typically translated as "the lotus flower"; it is actually a reference to the Egyptian blue water lily.[5] This flower appears in the book of Job:

> Behold the [hippopotamus] Behemoth! which I made along with you...what power... He ranks first among the works of God, yet his maker can approach him with a sword...Under the lotus plants [water lilies] he lies, hidden

4   Berlin and Brettler 2004, p.1500.
5   Emboden 1979; Seawright 2001.

among the reeds in the marsh. The lotuses [water lilies]
conceal him in their shadow...[6]

It might be easy to dismiss this passage as too obscure and
indecipherable because of its one-time use of words. However,
if we do so, we would miss obvious keys to decoding Job's
shamanic role and identity. In this passage, God not only
compares Job to the mythical Behemoth (Behema in Hebrew)—
the dangerous hippopotamus who sleeps under the shadow
of the water plants—but he also claims to have created them
at the same time. While this assertion appears to contradict
the sequence of creation reported in the Genesis story, it
serves to establish the essential unity and identity of Job
and the Behemoth. Job, hereby, is placed in the role of God's
adversary in the primordial battle (against Behemoth and
Leviathan[7]) through which God established the current order
of the universe. This contest echoes ancient Mesopotamian
and Near Eastern creation stories of the primeval world
battle to establish order over chaos. At the same time, Job
plays the role of God's assistant, helping God win the contest
against the Adversary. What sense is to be made of this double
identity that Job is made to play? What is the significance of
this ambivalence?

When we examine the role of Behemoth, the wild
hippopotamus, in ancient Egyptian mythology, we witness the
same double role as monster and helper in this single figure.
The hippopotamus appears in pre-dynastic Egyptian myth as
a helper to the hero or shaman as it makes its journey through
the dark underworld and then returns to life and light. Based
on the role of the midwife, the Goddess Tauret appears in

---

6   Job 40 (translation: Kohlenberger 1987).
7   Job 40-41.

the form of a hippopotamus. She assists in the daily rebirth and reappearance of Ra, the sun god, from the lotus in his solar travels.[8]

The Egyptians recognized Ra, the Sun god, in the blue water lily's ascent, as bringing the sun from underworld realms of death and darkness.[9] So, too, the ancient Greeks represented this same journey with Apollo, the solar charioteer and Lord of Delphi, who delivered the solar orb from its nightly captivity in underworld depths. The sun's journey—through the aromatic and visual symbolism of lotus and water lily—becomes an archetypal vehicle for shamanic voyaging.

When the hippopotamus is absorbed into later Egyptian religious belief, it undergoes a radical transformation into a powerful and dangerous monster, as does the Behemoth in the Bible. Thus, when Job is cited as being identical to the Behemoth, the underworld journey and shamanic identity are implicit in the reference to the shadowy water plant under which the biblical Behemoth hides.

PLANTS AND PURPOSE

The lotus was the supreme plant of the Egyptian repertoire of sacred plants, because of its fragrant scent, its alternating life course beneath and above the water, and its capacity to induce altered states of consciousness. While the story of Job is set on the shores of the Jordan River, the references to the lotus and the hippopotamus demonstrate that Egyptian myth, religion, and iconography were employed to tell this tale.

For the Egyptians, the scent of the plant—its essence—was the spirit of the deity. While the segments of the plant

8   Mercatante 1978.
9   Clark 1959.

represent the different parts of the gods' and goddesses' bodies, it is the scent that was the divine spirit itself. Worshipped as Nefertum, god of the Egyptian perfumers, this god of the sacred psychoactive lotus articulated this worship of scent as divine.

> I invoke Nefertum, in the following of Ptah. Thou art guardian and protector of the perfume and oil makers, protector and god of the sacred lotus. Osiris is the body of the plants. Nefertum is the soul of the plants, the plants purified. The divine perfume belongs to Nefertum living forever.[10]

Throughout ancient Egyptian art and iconography, the act of smelling the lotus is repeatedly depicted as the focus of the image.[11]

When the fragrant Egyptian lotus appears in the book of Job, it signifies spiritual descent and darkness. In this biblical context, this darkness is the home of the ferocious wild hippopotamus. Called a "shady tree," under which the hippopotamus dwells, the verse refers to the long stalk of the blue water lily (*Nymphaea caerulea*).[12] Its roots rest in the underwater mud while its flower ascends, untainted by the sludge from which it arises, into the morning sunlight in a cyclical process of ascent and descent.[13] In the book of Job, the focus is on this watery underworld interlude as a place of darkness and descent.

The psychoactive effects of blue water lily—alluded to in this description of the Behemoth and underwater darkness beneath the lotus (lily)—produce the mental significance

....

10   Lawless, 1994, p.49.
11   Manniche 1989.
12   Bertol *et al*. 2004; Seawright 2001.
13   Alexander 2015.

of the Behemoth's abode. Religious scholar William Emboden has convincingly re-examined the Egyptian iconography of the blue water lily.[14] Many of the scenes that were previously interpreted as mourning and mortuary are actually scenes of healing, demonstrating the medical use of blue water lily.[15] This hypnotic condition and the return from it into waking consciousness, as Emboden explains, is narrated as a journey. Hereby, the process of ascent and descent are the two parts of a single journey, but ascent is not necessarily assured. To return is the challenge of the shaman's journey.

Like the submerged hippopotamus, Job's shamanic journey through underworld regions must emerge from the hypnotic effects of the water lily into the clarity of aware consciousness. The text, then, presents the reader with a conundrum: the ultimate message that divine consciousness cannot be fathomed appears to contradict resolution. Though God reprimands Job for his need of an explanation for suffering, God also compensates him by demonstrating the awe and majesty of creation before Job's eyes. Even though the divine mind may not be able to be explained, in this way, it can be *experienced*. Accordingly, Job is blessed on his return with abundance, progeny, and wealth. His shamanic journey to conquer otherworldly challenges results in the redemption, healing, and affirmation of the unknowability of God.

How did this happen? Let's trace the pathway.

THE PSYCHOLOGY OF THE SHAMAN

Job's story follows the narrative framework of the shaman's archetypal otherworldly battle.

....

14   Emboden 1979, 1981, 1989.
15   Bertol *et al.* 2004; Harer 1985; Merlin 2003.

The shaman is defined as a cultural hero and healer who performs his healing by traveling to unseen worlds of the spirit—often through the agency of dreams, visions, altered states, or psychoactive plants—to rescue and redeem lost souls.[16] Job's calling came about through a dream vision:

> A word came to me in stealth;
> My ear caught a whisper of it.
> In thought-filled visions of the night,
> When deep sleep falls on men,
> Fear and trembling came upon me,
> Causing all my bones to quake with fright.
> A wind passed by me,
> Making the hair on my flesh bristle.
> It halted; its appearance was strange to me;
> A form loomed before my eyes;
> I heard a murmur and a voice...[17]

Whereas a shaman is summoned because of the disappearance of a person's soul or life spirit (proposed to have been abducted into the underworld by contesting spirits), Job must travel into unseen realms of consciousness to prove his faith. Along the way, a shaman meets friendly and helpful spirits as well as malevolent and destructive adversaries. It is the shaman's job to venture into that dangerous territory to battle terrifying monsters and to rescue that abducted soul or departed spirit.[18]

Specifically, Job's shamanic underworld journey is a battle of psychological transformation. It begins as an entry into a dark landscape of the mind and is manifested by

---

16 Eliade 1967; Siegel and Conquergood 1985, 1992; Conquergood and Paja Thao 1989; Halifax 1982; Shannon 2008.

17 Job 4.12-16 (translation and ascription of dream to Job rather than Eliphaz; Berlin and Brettler 2004).

18 Conquergood and Paja Thao 1989; Siegel and Conquergood 1985, 1992. New York: Filmakers Library.

physical illness and disability. This leads Job to the brink of "suicidal despair":[19]

> God damn the day I was born
> And the night that forced me from the womb.
> On that day let there be darkness...
> Why couldn't I have died as they
> pulled me out of the dark?[20]

Such is a test of the true shaman: can he defeat the darkness and survive to return to light, life, and the land of the living— even if those terrifying visions are created by none other than his own God:

> If I say, "My bed will comfort me,
> My couch will soothe my pain,"
> You frighten me with dreams
> And terrify me with visions[21]

THE JOURNEY OF THE EGYPTIAN BLUE WATER LILY AND THE RISKS OF RETURN

Healing is the goal of the shaman's journey and Job's mission is to heal the spiritual rupture of human and supernatural domains. Should the shaman fail in this netherworld battle, he surrenders to the dangerous waters never to return again—the healing mission thus failed in the realms of both the living and dead. That mythical voyage is also occurring on the psychological level through the psychoactive effects of the fragrant blue water lily. Ingestion of psychoactive plants always risk uncertain consequences and it is up to the skill of

---

19 Edinger 1986, p.29ff.
20 Job 3.3 (translation: Mitchell 1987).
21 ·Job 7.13-14.

the shaman to tread this dangerous path on behalf of those he rescues.

Homer's *Odyssey* offers a tale of the unsuccessful journey of a people called Lotus-Eaters. On an island between Troy and Ithaka, Odysseus's homeland, they represent the psychological risk of becoming stuck in the effects of the narcotic plant, never to return to their homeland or their waking awareness:

> I [Odysseus] was driven thence by foul winds for a space of nine days upon the sea, but on the tenth day we reached the land of the Lotus-eaters, who live on a food that comes from a kind of flower. Here we landed to take in fresh water...I sent two of my company to see what manner of men the people of the place might be, and they had a third man under them. They started at once, and went among the Lotus-eaters, who did them no hurt, but gave them to eat of the lotus, which was so delicious that those who ate of it left off caring about home, and did not even want to go back and say what happened to them, but were for staying and munching lotus with the Lotus-eaters without thinking further of their return; nevertheless, though they wept bitterly I forced them back to the ships and made them fast under the benches. Then I told the rest to go on board at once, lest any of them should taste of the lotus and leave off wanting to go home...[22]

This is Job's shamanic challenge: to successfully complete this journey and return to everyday consciousness.

Iconographically, the danger that the hippopotamus and the blue water lily represent is shown on blue faience hippopotami found in ancient Egyptian tombs of the Middle

---

22 Homer, *Odyssey*, Book 9.

Kingdom.[23] The (restored) feet of these figurines appear to have been intentionally broken as if to restrain the animal from attacking or fleeing, thereby uniting its role both as adversary or monster, and assistant or soul guide, during the dangerous underworld journey. Still, its hopeful aspect of renewal was consistently represented with the blossoming blue water lilies drawn on the back haunches of all 50 of the tomb figurines. Job, as the figurative Behemoth resting beneath the water lilies, necessarily carries all these associations in his narrative role as the protagonist in the battle between God and the Adversary.

THE THREE CHALLENGES

As Job enters conditions of darkness when divine and adversarial opponents battle out their positions by testing Job with three trials, Job is visited by three friends who challenge Job in three rounds. Three figures are standard characters in shamanic myths and folklore and represent the heroic challenges or riddles that the shaman must resolve to succeed in his mission.[24] We note the same configuration when Abraham was visited by three divine and prophetic persons during his time of disability. Like Abraham's divine guests, Job's friends give him a central question and prophetic message of his purpose, plot, and mission.

Each of Job's three visitors presents him with a repetition of staid traditional values and rigid religious logic. These are challenges to Job's perception, interpretation, and construction of a new and integrated meaning of his condition. Should he agree with any of these values that too easily resolve

....
23 Metropolitan Museum of Art 1917.
24 Ruck *et al.* 2007.

his conundrum, Job will have failed on his journey. As biblical scholar Damon explains, Job's "finding of the true God is also the finding of his own true individuality...Job's disasters are not punitive, but educational. They rouse Job from his complacent submissiveness to tradition, and start him on his search for his true God."[25]

As the tale of the Lotus-Eaters demonstrates, failure translates into a stalled journey, which results in the inability to return to life and home. Job must reject all these explanations to achieve a higher and more complex understanding of the interaction of human and divine consciousnesses. When a new personality—Elihu, meaning "my God [is] Lord"—appears in the text and reveals the future, we are narratively and symbolically assured that Job has successfully survived. The story ultimately culminates with Job's acceptance of the unknowability of divine consciousness. Job's stalwart position of innocence against the blame of his friends will be confirmed and affirmed by divine punishment of those friends for their harassment of Job. In this way, Job serves to validate divine consciousness in his insistence on innocence and faith.

The final scene where Job's losses—family, property, wealth, health, etc.—are restored in a manner that is even more beautiful and resplendent than before indicates that those institutions, of family, society, and religion themselves also were in need of healing. The deficiency they represented is countered at the story's end by God's restoration of those institutions with greater depth and meaning.

Job's successful journey is signaled by another set of three. The naming of his children indicates a particular understanding of the story's resolution. As translator and scholar Stephen Mitchell points out, Job's seven sons and three

....
25 Damon 1966, pp.6-7.

61

daughters are nameless at the start of the story. This is not so at the end of the tale. There, Job's seven new sons remain nameless, while his three new daughters are given specific names: Dove, Cassia, and Kohl (eye-liner). Rather than being a random or arbitrary list, their names celebrate the renewed values that Job has achieved. Those values center around the sustaining experiences of culture: the dove of peaceful existence, the aromatic cassia that is a fragrant ingredient of sacred incense and religious worship, and beauty (of the female face). Additionally, these daughters are given equal share with the sons in Job's inheritance.

Job reveals that he has achieved a dual awareness; though unknowable, the mind of God may be experienced and embodied by the shaman who pursues truth and meaning against its opposite. Through this paradox of maintaining contradiction—that is, the divine is unknowable yet able to be experienced—Job demonstrates the successful psychological and spiritual journey whereby consciousness is expanded and awareness enlarged. Secure now in his successful underworld voyage and shamanic standing, Job earns and achieves the direct vision of God:

> I have heard you with my ears;
> But now I see you with my eyes...[26]

While in the end Job's witness to God's truth is demonstrated by Job's renewed and generous blessings of family and wealth, Job ultimately answers humanity's most pressing existential question about the mind of God. Thereby, health, well-being, and order are restored to the individual and to his community through the shaman's physical and metaphysical journey.

....

26 Job 42.5 (translation: Berlin and Brettler 2004).

CONCLUSION

Job's ultimate understanding rejects simplistic explanations of his suffering and fate. Instead, Job comes to the conclusion that, in fact, divine consciousness is unknowable. Human consciousness is incomplete and fragmented. With this conclusion, the ambivalence and ambiguity that arose throughout the reading of this passage come to contribute to this understanding and experience of the ineffability of divine consciousness. Throughout the tale, the reader is presented with irreconcilable inconsistencies— for example, the shaman as helper *and* as adversary—that prepare the reader to accept this outcome. Unsatisfying as the conclusion of the inscrutability of the Unknown may be, it is actually the only satisfying outcome to Job's suffering as Job himself concludes. The ambivalences that pervade the text shape the narrative experience of the reader, creating an encounter with and an acceptance of the undefined, contradictory, and multivalent workings of the universe. Synchronously, the text insists that the divine can be experienced through the senses. Through this awareness, Job is named "the greatest of the men of the East" (Job 1.3).

As a model for contemporary healing practices, the story of Job offers much to consider. By highlighting the role of the fragrant plant that motivates and shapes the psychological journey, the aromatic healer today is given a model of change and transformation that is implicit and necessary in the healing process. Rather than assuming an immediate and narrative-free experience of suffering and its cure, the healer assumes the role of the shaman who facilitates a story of journeying through the darkness of pain and suffering into the clarity of meaning and light. In the chapters that follow this first examination of the book of Job as prototype for the role of the healer as shaman, I explore diverse aromatic plants and narratives that achieve the healing state.

BIBLIOGRAPHY

Alexander, R. (2015) Personal correspondence. Plant Answer Line Librarian of the Elizabeth C. Miller Library, University of Washington, USA.

Berlin, A. and Brettler, M.Z. (2004) *The Jewish Study Bible*. Oxford: Oxford University Press.

Bertol, E., Fineschi, V., Karch, S.B., Mari, F., and Riezzo, I. (2004) "*Nymphaea* cults in ancient Egypt and the New World: a lesson in empirical pharmacology." *Journal of the Royal Society of Medicine 97*, 2, 84-85.

Clark, R.T. (1959) *Myth and Symbol in Ancient Egypt*. London: Thames & Hudson.

Conquergood, D. and Paja Thao (1989) *I Am a Shaman: A Hmong Life Story with Ethnographic Commentary*. Minneapolis, MN: Center for Urban and Regional Affairs, University of Minnesota.

Damon, S.F. (1966) *Blake's Job: William Blake's Illustrations of the Book of Job*. Providence, RI: Brown University Press.

Edinger, E. (1986) *Encounter with the Self: A Jungian Commentary on William Blake's Illustrations of the Book of Job*. Toronto: Inner City Books.

Eliade, M. (1967) *Shamanism: Archaic Techniques of Ecstasy*. Princeton, NJ: Princeton University Press.

Emboden, W. (1978) "Sacred Narcotic Water Lily of the Nile: *Nymphaea caerulea*." *Economic Botany 33*, 1, 395-407.

Emboden, W. (1981)"Transcultural use of narcotic water lilies in ancient Egyptian and Maya drug ritual." *Journal of Ethnopharmacology 3*, 1, 39-83.

Emboden, W. (1989) "The sacred journey in dynastic Egypt: shamanistic trance in the context of the narcotic water lily and mandrake." *Journal of Psychoactive Drugs 21*, 1, 61-75.

Fadiman, A. (1997) *The Spirit Catches You and You Fall Down: A Hmong Child, Her American Doctors, and the Collision of Two Cultures*. New York: Farrar, Strauss and Giroux.

Halifax, J. (1982) *Shaman: The Wounded Healer*. London: Thames & Hudson.

Harer, W.B. (1985) "Pharmacological and biological properties of the Egyptian lotus." *Journal of the American Research Center in Egypt 22*, 49-54.

Jacob, I. and Jacob, W. (1992) "Water Plants—Water Lily." In D.N. Freedman (ed.) *The Anchor Bible Dictionary*. New York: Doubleday.

Kohlenberger III, J.R. (1987) *The Interlinear NIV Hebrew-English Old Testament*. Grand Rapids, MI: Zondervan Publishing House.

Lawless, J. (1994) *Aromatherapy and the Mind*. San Francisco, CA: Thorsons.

Manniche, L. (1989) *An Ancient Egyptian Herbal*. Austin, TX: University of Texas Press.

Mercatante, A. (1978) *Who's Who in Egyptian Mythology*. New York: Clarkson N. Potter.

Merlin, M. (2003) "Archaeological evidence for the tradition of psychoactive plant use in the Old World." *Economic Botany 57*, 3, 295-323.

Metropolitan Museum of Art (1917) "An Egyptian hippopotamus figure." *Bulletin of the Metropolitan Museum of Art 4*, 78.

Mitchell, S. (1987) *The Book of Job*. New York: HarperPerennial.

Pope, M. (1973) *The Anchor Bible: Job*. New York: Doubleday.

Ruck, C.A.P., Staples, B.D., Gonzalez, J.A., and Hoffman, M.A. (2007) *The Hidden World Survival of Pagan Shamanistic Themes in European Fairytales*. Durham, NC: Carolina Academic Press.

Scheindlin, R. (1998) *The Book of Job*. New York: W.W. Norton.

Seawright, C. (2001) "The Egyptian 'Lotus'—Nymphaea Caerulea, The Blue Water Lily." Egyptology. Available at www.thekeep. org/~kunoichi/kunoichi/themestream/egypt_waterlily.html#. WHp4dxBMR8V, accessed on January 17, 2017.

Shannon, B. (2008) "Biblical entheogens: a speculative hypothesis." *Time and Mind: The Journal of Archaeology, Consciousness, and Culture 1*, 1, 51-74.

Siegel, T. and Conquergood, D. (1985) *Between Two Worlds: The Hmong Shaman in America*. Video recording. Alexandria, VA: Filmakers Library.

Siegel, T. and Conquergood, D. (1992) *The Heart Broken in Half*. Video recording. New York: Filmakers Library.

Winkelman, M. (2004) "Shamanism as the original neurotheology." *Zygon 39*, 1, 193-217.

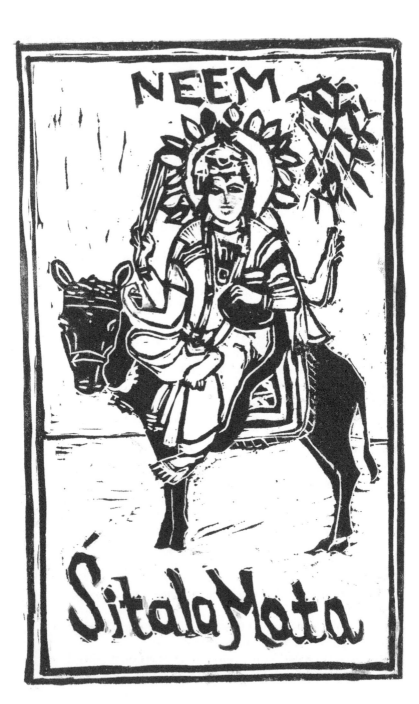

CHAPTER 3

TO NEEM OR NOT

*On the Benefits of Ambivalence and the Worship
of the Hindu Smallpox Goddess Sitala Mata*

INTRODUCTION

The neem tree (*Azadirachta indica*) represents one of the clearest examples of the achievement and experience of paradoxical consciousness as a healing state. During one of the most intense historical periods of epidemic in India—the smallpox epidemic—the Hindu goddess, Sitala Mata, personification of the neem tree, who presided over the sick beds of the ill, was both creator of the disease and its cure. In addition, the sick person was believed to embody the goddess in the experience of smallpox.

This paradox represents and renders an existential crisis that is embodied in the neem tree, *Azadirachta indica* (*margosa* in Sanskrit). It concerns the Hindu goddess Sitala Mata, the avatar and personification of the neem tree. The crisis centers on the nature of her identity. Is she solely a goddess of disease, specifically poxes and fevers? Or, is she the goddess, the Mata or Mother, of healing those diseases? Both identities conspire to place her at the "scene of the crime"; that is, at the bedside and altar of the sick. Thus, her identity is crucial to our understanding of healing with potent plants, such as neem.

The study of Sitala Mata beliefs and rituals offers us valuable insights by inviting us to consider the patient as more than a set of symptoms and ailments to be treated. Instead, we are put on a quest for human wholeness. This inquiry into the identity of Sitala Mata and her neem tree offers us a model that integrates previously rejected aspects of self into a greater unity. An integrated identity is the definition and goal of health. Hereby, an inquiry into the dual identity of Sitala Mata provides us with a framework for examining the dimensions of an integrated self. It also offers us the means to identify the disability of a "divided self" for use in aromatic healing today. Neem represents this effort to imagine and to construct the unified self.

THE SMALLPOX GODDESS

A folk goddess, Sitala Mata was integrated into later Hinduism and her worship persisted in her domain over poxes, fevers, and skin diseases even after smallpox was eradicated in 1977 by the collaboration between the Indian government and the World Health Organization (WHO). Smallpox was spread by person to person contact, through contaminated clothing and objects, and by airborne water droplets conveyed from human host to the next human host, only ending when the human chain of victims ceased. Hereby, smallpox quickly became an epidemic.[1] Smallpox produced painful and scarring

1   Hopkins 1983, p.10.

pustules mainly on the face, trunk, hands, and feet, an intense fever, and possible blindness. Before vaccinations became available, smallpox was highly contagious and oftentimes it was deadly, killing over half a million people during the duration of the epidemic.[2]

Jenner's development of a smallpox vaccination in 1796 enabled its final eradication in India and the world in 1977. However, we cannot ignore the folk method that preceded Jenner's vaccination by at least 200 years, if not more.[3] Called *variolation* after the smallpox virus (*variola major*), it was made by drying the scabs of infected patients or lancing their boils and using these products to "variolate" or inoculate a patient. Perhaps this protective procedure is what inspires the paradoxical identity of the goddess. By taking in the disease, the patient becomes protected from the disease. What made Jenner's vaccination so effective, surpassing the variolation technique, was its method of administration. By immunizing all the people in a wide circle around the infected patient, a circle of containment was created, thereby interrupting and breaking the chain of smallpox transmission.

Sitala Mata, whose name means "the cool one" or "the cooling one," is a mother (*mata*) goddess whose worship focused on the illness and curing of smallpox. Smallpox induced intense fevers and so Sitala Mata's command of coolness was her defining feature. The patient with smallpox was served "cool" drinks and "cooled" foods, and the entire household followed these ritual prohibitions against warmth: no fried or hot foods were consumed, no cooking allowed, and no "heated" interactions, arguments, or

....

2   Davis 2015; Henderson 2009.

3   Hopkins 1983, p.17.

disagreements permitted. Anger represented the rage of the goddess manifest in outbreaks of smallpox.

> Suffering from the disease can be spoken of in terms of an excess of heat, the pustules being the visible sign of an overboiling blood erupting through the skin and the fever the immediate indication of an excess of heat escaping from the body. It can also and simultaneously be spoken of as the anger of the goddess... Anger is an excess of heat...[4]

Through cleanliness and adherence to the ritual prohibitions, the patient invites the goddess to renounce her feverish rage (heat).

Iconography of Sitala Mata offers clues for decipherment of her existential meaning. She is represented in statuary and paintings as riding on a donkey and carrying a water bowl, a broom, a pot, and a winnowing fan or a bunch of neem leaves. The donkey, an animal known to suffer from pronounced boils, thereby demonstrating its physical association with the disease,[5] is the goddess's vehicle, literally and metaphorically. Sitala Mata carries in her hands the tools of her healing practice. All display the ambivalence and ultimate unity of disease and its cure. The broom sweeps in dual directions, the winnowing fan separates material into distinct forms, the pot of virus pulses is evidence of disease that is used for inoculations against disease, and the water bowl and neem leaves provide the healing dimensions of cooling waters and medicinal plants that signal the triumph over fever and illness and the return to wholeness. The traumatic devastation and brutal deaths that smallpox produced ensured the persistence of memory even after the eradication of the disease. Worship of

4   Marglin 1987, p.17.
5   Ferrari 2015.

Sitala Mata persevered and continues today. Cornelia Davis, a WHO physician who worked with the Indian smallpox eradication program, explains: "Sitala Mata always needs to be appeased so that her wrath doesn't bring on other epidemics."[6]

NEEM, HEALING, AND THE PARADOX OF PLAY

In neem healing practice, the suffering person is bathed in cool neem-infused waters and rests on a bed lined with aromatic neem leaves.[7] The patient is rubbed with neem leaves as prayers to the goddess are recited. A neem branch is waved over the patient to provide a cooling breeze and it is said to be the voice of Sitala Mata who speaks through its fluttering leaves. With the release of its volatile oils through the waving of the leaves, the scent heralds the arrival and presence of the goddess. Oftentimes not appreciated by "Western noses" and found to be disagreeable, the scent of neem is considered "refreshing" and pleasant by most Hindus.[8] She is the invigorating and powerful smell of neem. The goddess inspires dream visions through the whispering of the scented neem leaves.[9] Ultimately, through ritual and its employment of neem, the goddess provides caring for her suffering devotee.

An evergreen tree native to India, neem currently grows throughout southern Asia in tropical and subtropical climates. Its healing properties and potencies are wide ranging: it is anti-inflammatory, antipyretic, fungicidal,

6   Davis 2015, p.224.
7   Conrick 2009; Mukhopadhyay 1994.
8   My thanks to Sravanyi Bhattacharjee for this insight.
9   Ferrari 2015.

antihistamine, and antiseptic. These properties are produced by two main triterpenoids: azadirachtin and nimbin that are found in all parts of the tree: roots, bark, leaves, wood, and oil.[10] Neem has been hailed as an agrarian savior of the underdeveloped world by international organizations. The United Nations Development and Environment Programs cite the neem tree as the "Tree of the 21st Century." The United States National Academy of Science, similarly, identifies Neem as "Neem: A Tree for Solving Global Problems"[11] and the WHO calls it a "wonder tree."[12] Hindu mythology also recognized these seemingly miraculous potencies of the neem tree. The neem tree was said to gain its curative powers when, at the beginning of time, the primeval great Lord Indra was carrying a golden goblet of the magical amrita (ambrosia) liquid—the elixir of immortality—to the realm of the gods when some of the liquid spilled from the bowl and splashed onto the neem tree below it. That is the source of the amazing power of neem according to traditional sources.

Clearly, neem's antiviral, antipyretic, and antiseptic potencies were useful and important in avoiding and in treating the symptoms of smallpox. Religious rituals in honor of the goddess of smallpox, Sitala Mata, display therapeutic methods of disease management employing neem. As WHO educator S.H. Hassan explains, "many of these rural songs [to Sitala Mata] have health education values which was never realized by the health staff...cleanliness when there is a case of smallpox..."[13] Remarkably, songs to Sitala Mata narrate therapeutic procedures.[14] In these performances, the

10   Kraus 1995; Puri 1999; Singh *et al.* 2009.
11   National Research Council 1992.
12   Kumar and Navaratnam 2013.
13   Hassan 1977, p.4.
14   Hassan 1977; Wadley 1980.

patient embodies the goddess and enacts her part in the drama of illness. Although the giving of smallpox variolations and vaccinations could have challenged, or even threatened, the ritual model, vaccinations were normalized by bringing them into the context of Sitala Mata worship. For example, the following song was sung at an inoculation administration; the patient *is* the goddess, addressed as Sitalamayya (Mother Sitala).

> Sitalamayya plays and dances in a circle on a clean courtyard and on clean paths. While dancing and playing in a circle, Sitalmayyya [perspires]

> Bhairav, please bring flower fan and a bough of Neem for Sitalmayya.

> Q. Bhairavi says, "O Mother, from where shall I bring flower fan, from where shall I bring bough of Neem?

> A. (Sitalmayya answers): Bring flower fan from the gardener's shop and Neem bough from the forest.

> Q. Mother, who will fan you with flower fan, who will fan you with the bough of Neem?

> A. Mother of child (having smallpox) will fan me with flower fan and Bjahta (servant of Goddess) will fan me with bough of neem.[15]

The process of attending to the sick (or vaccinated patient) is seen as service to Sitala Mata. After 14 days, the vaccinator returns to the home of the patient to perform the ritual of "Nimaiah Puja," the worship of the neem tree.[16]

....

15 Hassan 1977, p.4.
16 Hassan 1977, p.4.

As we witness, these rituals reveal a particular attitude and identification between Sitala and her patient. Hindu scholar Fabrizio Ferrari named it "possession."[17] In these songs to the smallpox goddess Sitala Mata, and in practice, we see a total identification on the part of the patient with the goddess. The patient *is* Sitala Mata, experiencing her needs and expressing the healing process of the ritual procedure. As Frédérique Marglin explains:

> Treating the patient and worshiping the goddess are one and the same set of actions and words. The diseased person male or female is addressed as "mother" (ma); he or she is offered cooling drinks and food, leaves of the neem tree which are said to be cooling as well as being a disinfecting agent. In other words, the patient is offered the same substances which the goddess might simultaneously be offered in her temple, as well as being spoken of and to as if he or she were the goddess herself.[18]

Smallpox and her other diseases were spoken of as Sitala Mata's "play" in the human realm. Thus, the person suffering from smallpox was considered to be the goddess, who plays in the human realm through the bodies of her devotees, and treated accordingly. As David Arnold explains:

> Although Sitala is often referred to as "the goddess of smallpox" or simply "the smallpox goddess," smallpox was understood to be a manifestation of her personality and presence rather than her essential character. The disease was her "sport" or "play" and had to be tolerated accordingly or given the respect and honor due to the

---

17 Ferrrari 2010; 2015; Brosius and Husken 2010.
18 Marglin 1987, p.17.

visiting goddess...her entry into the body demanded ritual rather than therapeutic responses.[19]

Through total identification with the goddess, the patient experienced that play as possession by the goddess, thereby erasing the boundaries between Self and Other. The participants then bid farewell to Sitala in the same manner as that by which they bid farewell to a newly married bride about to travel to her new home. Sitala's "play" was completed with the worship of the Neem tree. Whether the disease and its treatment ran their courses, or the disease was pre-empted through the vaccination that was incorporated into traditional worship, both methods recognized that the goddess Sitala Mata was in charge.

EMBRACING AMBIVALENCE

Sitala Mata is embodied in the neem tree that is adorned and worshipped as the incarnation of the goddess.[20] Neem trees typically are planted outside of Sitala Mata's temples. To grow a Neem tree outside one's home is a sign of great blessing. Used for a tremendous variety of illnesses and conditions, neem is the appropriate expression of the beneficent Mata (Mother) Goddess. The love and respect that the Hindus proffer the Neem tree is both tangible and metaphysical. It demonstrates the capacity of the natural world to "absorb" suffering through its gifts of healing.

It is believed that trees have an enormous capacity to absorb suffering, since they have an abundance of auspiciousness, goodwill, and generosity. As part of the

19 Arnold 1993, pp.122–123.
20 Haberman 2013.

greater natural world, their sacredness is naturally more encompassing than that of humans...the tree will bear the burden of human suffering, and, in a sense, transform the suffering and inauspiciousness into auspiciousness... is another example of embedded ecologies.[21]

At the same time, the neem tree is believed to go through the process of human pain and ambivalence. Thus, pregnant women treat the neem tree with whatever medicines and treatments that they are using—as if the neem is a sort of Other or surrogate in the birthing process.[22] Some see this as anthropomorphizing the natural world, thereby subsuming nature as human self. From this perspective, the small bronze face masks and red saris that adorn neem trees to demonstrate their identity as the goddess Sitala might throw us into a dangerous and fruitless opposition between Self and Other (that I discuss shortly). Other scholars, however, do not project that anthropomorphic meaning onto the human face masks on the neem trees. David Haberman, accordingly, cites their use to facilitate and establish mutual *relationship*. Thereby, the projected self (face mask) onto the other (neem tree) represents a process of unity and identification between sentient beings.

Sitala Mata, the embodiment of the divinity of neem, offers us a compelling model whereby disease and the healing of disease resides within a single being. This is an "ambivalent" identity—that is, it holds antithetical, contradictory, paradoxical, and rejected significances simultaneously. Thus, as a neem tree goddess, Sitala Mata's leaves are used to mark the home where contagious disease, such as pox and

....
21 Nagarajan 2000, p.459; Haberman 2013, p.159; Chapple and Tucker 2000.
22 Karthikeyan 2012.

fever, is present. At the same time, neem leaves and oils are employed in the treatment and healing of the disease. This approach is emotionally and spiritually unifying because it avoids the psychological splitting that Freud identified as the origin of ill health: "The inability to tolerate ambiguity is the origin of neurosis."[23] The goddess Sitala Mata both causes and cures disease in what we may consider a dialectical expression of unified identity. Moniker-Williams, writing in 1879, recognized this multifaceted valence of the figure of Sitala who is "the mother who presides over small-pox, and may prevent small-pox, cause small-pox, or be herself small-pox."[24]

This paradoxical unification of possible identities has implications for understandings of health and illness beyond the specifics of smallpox. It refers to:

> the indigenous Indian (folk and Ayurvedic particularly) notion of disease as an imbalance between a variety of factors, none of which should or could be expelled or eradicated. Thus health is not understood as an absence of disease but as a state of harmonious congruence between humors in the body and between these and their corresponding elements in the natural, social, and cosmological environment.[25]

In other words, Sitala Mata represents extremes that must be brought into balance to achieve health.

Sitala Mata is inherently ambivalent, as we witness in the divergent academic assessments of her smallpox identity and her cure. Ferrari, a scholar of Hindu religion, claims that the exclusive focus on Sitala Mata as a goddess of

....

23 Freud (source unknown).
24 Quoted in Ferrari 2010, p.147.
25 Marglin 1987, p.25.

disease is the outcome of distorted, prejudicial, and colonial interpretations of the evidence of her worship.

> Representations of Sitala have suffered from uncritical (and partial) readings of Indian texts. They also have been affected by colonial and post-colonial agendas... All these aspects converge in the rendering of Sitala as a "disease goddess" rather than healing mother...[26]

Ferrari explains the result is to neglect the antithetical position of proclaiming that Sitala is "a benevolent Mother and goddess of hygiene"[27] that is implicit in *bhakti* (devotional) worship. However, we must resist going to the opposite extreme whereby we are compelled to take an either/or interpretive stance, such as *either* she is a destructive disease goddess as colonialist interpreters claim, *or* she is a beneficent healing mother. By not proposing an understanding of the paradoxical unity and ambivalence of these twin identities, we risk falling into a divided and dissonant state of mind. In other words, by separating Sitala Mata's identity into dichotomized and irreconcilable extremes, we are repeating what Freud charged as the impetus for the slide into disability through the inability to tolerate ambivalence.

Splitting Sitala Mata into irreconcilable poles of good and bad has psychological consequences. It mandates identification with one extreme and rejects the other as alien. In this act, the accepted self is idealized and divested of any negativity and, as a consequence, the rejected pole is vilified. We see this easily, for example, with the contemporary splitting of women's personas into dualistic sexual stereotypes.[28] Such polarization fails to capture the complexity and ambiguity of the lived lives

26 Ferrari 2015, p.xx.
27 Ferrari 2015, p.xix.
28 Denmark and Paludi 1993; Freud 1912.

of women—or goddesses. Scholar of Hinduism Wendy Doniger explains that polarization is evidence of a sexually oppressive system. She cites the multiplicity of Hindu goddesses as expression of a less rigid system of belief and practice, and as evidence of alternative models of integration.[29]

The mythology of neem provides us with a model for thinking about healing, its requirements and practices. For example, contemporary consumer-capitalist culture inculcates an identity of narcissistic entitlement in its participants.[30] Necessarily, narcissistic entitlement requires the polarization of emotions and identity to exist. "All about me," the claim of the entitled, not only focuses on the self as the single legitimate identity, but, also, in doing so, projects any negativity onto the polarized Other. The narcissistic Self, then, is idealized, without anything to balance or to challenge its supremacy.

This is a dangerous role to assume for the entitled Self and also for the rejected Other. Both come to be one-dimensional parodies without the complexity and subtlety of an integrated self. What the image of Sitala Mata compels us to consider is the necessity of seeking that integration. We cannot ignore or deny the power of the goddess to inflict disease, nor can we fail to acknowledge the healing powers over which she also presides. It is her "play." Accordingly, this integration is the "awe" that Sitala is said to inspire in her devotees. The path toward this psychological integration is, I believe, represented in her iconography as the symbolic tools for healing. We must, as the iconography of Sitala displays, be able to "hold" illness in our hands as we "ride" the disease and its process into wholeness.

....

29 Doniger 1999.
30 Robbins 2010.

THE DIVINE TREE

In aromatic healing, essential oils deriving from trees, such as neem, cedar, cypress, and pine, are oftentimes used to address concerns of the emotions, identity, and body. The tree hereby stands in symbolic and metaphorical relationship to the self. According to ancient Hindu belief, the tree, the divine, and the human share an existential identity. Manu (1.49), the ancient chronicler of religious law, states this expressly: "All trees and plants are full of consciousness within themselves and are endowed with the feelings of pleasure and pain."[31]

This recognition that both pleasure and pain are an integral part of life and cannot be separated is celebrated annually at New Year in India as the sign of balance and integration. A mixture of neem and *jagary* (raw sugar) is served and eaten— the bitter neem with sweet sugar reminds the celebrant that life is bittersweet (not one extreme or the other, but both together), a mixture represented by opposing tastes that are consumed together.[32]

The neem tree is more than the spatial location or residence of the goddess; the tree is the goddess herself. Certainly, aromatherapy today is used to address spiritual needs and deficiencies, oftentimes through essential oils from trees, but it is rare in Western experience to worship the tree itself as divine. Recent ecological studies concerning our relationship with the natural word and its maintenance would suggest that we would do well to reconsider and to redefine a troubled world-self to reclaim it as divine and to seek its healing.[33]

31 Olivelle 2004.
32 Thanks to Swami Yogatmananda for this information.
33 Weintrobe 2013.

CONCLUSION

With the necessity to balance the goddess's powers to cause and to cure disease, the ill patients and their caretakers are compelled to face the unknown, thereby requiring confrontation with fear, particularly fear of death and dying. Thus, Sitala's healing domain extended beyond disease into existential concerns. Her worship persists today throughout India, due in part to her capacity to provide this framework to achieve existential integration. With this goal of understanding in mind, we consider certain tree rituals from India that reveal important psychological and symbolic modes of healing that are relevant to aromatherapy today. Ambivalence poses a conundrum that must be addressed. By not assuming or expecting a singular totality—of person, time, space, emotions, or experience—the capacity to hold multiple identities and discordant narratives simultaneously is strengthened. Like Sitala Mata who holds the capacity both to cure and to cause disease, we seek that profound balance in understanding for healing. Certainly, a healing practice assumes that we not only accept shifting and changing identities—that is the goal of the work—but strive to enable that multiplicity and contradiction to be revealed, understood, and, ultimately, to be embraced.

BIBLIOGRAPHY

Arnold, D. (1993) *Colonizing the Body: State Medicine and Epidemic Disease in Nineteenth Century India*. Berkeley, CA: University of California Press.

Brosius, C. and Husken, U. (eds) (2010) *Ritual Matters: Dynamic Dimensions in Practice*. New York: Routledge.

Chapple, C.K. and M.E. Tucker (2000) *Hinduism and Ecology: The Intersection of Earth, Sky, and Water*. Cambridge, MA: Center for the Study of World Religions, Harvard University.

Conrick, J. (2009) *Neem: The Ultimate Herb*. Twin Lakes, WI: Lotus Press.

Davis, C. (2015) *Searching for Sitala: Eradicating Smallpox in India*. Laredo, TX: Konjit Publications.

Denmark, F. and Paludi, M. (1993) *A Psychology of Women: A Handbook of Issues and Theories*. Westport, CT: Greenwood Press.

Doniger, W. (1999) *Splitting the Difference: Gender and Myth in Ancient Greece and India*. Chicago: The University of Chicago Press.

Ferrari, F.M. (2010) "Old Rituals for New Threats: Possession and Healing in the Cults of Sitala." In C. Brosius and U. Husken (eds) *Ritual Matters: Dynamic Dimensions in Practice*. New York: Routledge.

Ferrari, F.M. (2015) *Religion, Devotion and Medicine in North India: The Healing Power of Sitala*. London: Bloomsbury.

Freud, S. (1912) "Uber die allgemeinste Emiedrigung des Liebeslebends" [the most prevalent form of degradation in erotic life]. In *Jahrbuch fur psychoanalytische und psychopathologische Forschungen 4*, 40-50.

Haberman, D. (2013) *People Trees: Worship of Trees in Northern India*. Oxford: Oxford University Press.

Hassan, S.H. (1977) "Farewell to Sitala Mayya." Geneva: World Health Organization.

Henderson, D.A. (2009) *Smallpox: The Death of a Disease*. Amherst, NY: Prometheus Books.

Hopkins, D.R. (1983) *The Greatest Killer: Smallpox in History*. Chicago: The University of Chicago Press.

Karthikeyan, A. (2012) "Heal with Neem." *The Hindu*, April 22.

Kraus, W. (1995) "Biologically Active Ingredients—Azadirachtin and Other Triterpenoids." In H. Schutterer (ed.) *The Neem Tree Azadirachta indica A. Juss and Other Meliaceous Plants*. New York: Weinheim, pp.35-88.

Kumar, V.S. and Navaratnam, V. (2013) "Neem (Azadirachta indica): Prehistory to contemporary medicinal uses to humankind." *Asian Pacific Journal of Tropical Biomedicine 3*, 7, 505-514.

Marglin, F.A. (July 1987) "Smallpox in Two Systems of Knowledge." Prepared for the UNU/WIDER Planning Meeting on Knowledge as Systems of Domination.

Mukhopadhyay, S.K. (1994) *Cult of Goddess Sitala in Bengal: An Inquiry into Folk Culture*. Calcutta: Firma KLM Private Limited.

Nagarajan, V. (2000) "Rituals of Embedded Ecologies: Drawing Kolams, Marrying Trees, and Generating Auspiciousness." In C.K. Chapple and M.E. Tucker (eds) *Hinduism and Ecology*. Cambridge, MA: Harvard University Press, pp.458-459.

National Research Council (1992) *Neem: A Tree for Solving Global Problems*. Washington, DC: National Academy Press.

Olivelle, P. (2004) *The Law of Manu*. New York: OUP.

Puri, H.S. (1999) *Neem: The Divine Tree. Azadirachta indica*. Amsterdam: Harwood Academic Publications.

Robbins, R. (2010) *Global Problems and the Culture of Capitalism*. New York: Pearson.

Singh, K.K., Phogat, S., Tomar, A., and Dhillon, R.S. (2009) *Neem: A Treatise*. New Delhi: International Publishing House.

Wadley, S. (1980) "Sitala: The Cool One." *Asian Folklore Studies 39*, 33-62.

Weintrobe, S. (ed.) (2013) *Engaging with Climate Change: Psychoanalytic and Interdisciplinary Perspectives*. New York: Routledge.

Yogatmananda (October 2014) Personal communication. Vedanta Society of Providence, RI, USA.

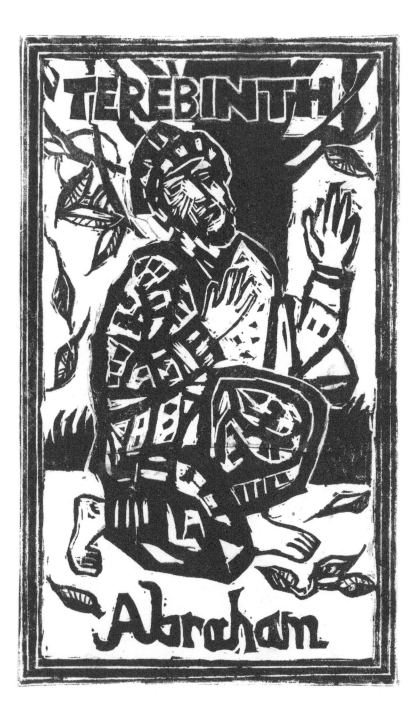

CHAPTER 4

THE FRAGRANCE OF TEREBINTH

A Fresh Look at the Ancient Akedah

*And they have built the shrines...to burn
their sons and daughters in the fire—*

which I never commanded, which never came to My mind...

JEREMIAH 7.31

INTRODUCTION

Terebinth (*Pistacia terebinthus*) propels us into profound questioning of existing frameworks of knowledge. It also reveals how the aromatic entry opens areas of understanding and insight that were previously unavailable. Specifically, this chapter explores the effects of terebinth as aromatic and metaphorical catalyst in the story of Abraham's development of a new religion and how it is embodied in three episodes in the biblical text. Terebinth induces a change of consciousness whereby Abraham is able to gain radical insight to envision a new spiritual reality. Through the breath, terebinth expands consciousness and provides the inspiration (literally, "the breathing in") for Abraham's insight. By this means, his altered cognition first appears as a dream, indicating that Abraham has achieved a higher level of awareness, but not that he is acting outside of time and space.

Sarah's laughter and impregnation continue this theme of inspiration. Laughter, the sudden expulsion of breath in the context of joy, defines and matches Abraham's terebinth inhalation. Moreover, laughter signals emotional and psychological release and so indicates the resolution of the dilemma that will culminate in the near sacrifice of Isaac. This chapter then re-examines the story of the binding of Isaac or Akedah through which Abraham articulates the dimensions of the religion he proposes. Abraham must introduce and normalize his new religion as distinct from existing Canaanite rites which are also held under terebinth trees.

TEREBINTH AND BREATH

While scholars recognize the "oracular and teaching" powers of the terebinth trees at Moreh and Mamre where the biblical Abraham meets his god,[1] scholars have neglected to examine the medicinal and spiritual properties of the essential oil of the terebinth tree as an actual and symbolic source of Abraham's heightened consciousness. These essential oil healing potencies of the biblical terebinth tree offer us a unique entry for understanding core concerns of the biblical text.

Producing a fragrant resinous gum, terebinth (*Pistacia terebinthus*) derives "from the incisions in the tree trunk [where] there flows a sort of transparent balsam, constituting a very pure and fine species of turpentine, with an agreeable odor, like citron or jessamine, and a mild taste, and hardening gradually into a transparent gum"[2] It acts as an analgesic,

1   Berlin and Brettler 2004, p.91.
2   McClintock and Strong 1981, pp.283–284.

antiseptic, rubefacient, and respiratory aid. Through inhalation, terebinth clears respiratory passageways and increases oxygen absorption, thereby enabling enhanced concentration and mental states of well-being.[3] God created the first human in the divine image by "breathing into his nostrils,"[4] designating the breath as the essence of divine consciousness.[5] Through breath, the fragrant oils of terebinth transform consciousness. The "terebinth is a bridge between human and divine spheres, and it becomes an arena of divine-human encounter, an ideal medium of oracles and revelation."[6]

The use of terebinth traces back to the Mediterranean Bronze Age in Minoan Crete.[7] Its name—with the characteristic "-nth" spelling—testifies to its pre-Indo-European origin. Archaeologist Sabine Beckmann has identified the terebinth tree in sacred seals of ritual worship.[8] Minoan iconography displays the terebinth tree as medium and method of otherworldly travel—both its goal and its promise of return. Representations in Minoan iconography reveal that the terebinth tree was esteemed as a visionary plant that originates in watery realms, resting beyond symbolic boundaries of waking consciousness. The Minoans, hereby, recognized and worshiped the divine origins of the terebinth tree.[9]

With such potencies, terebinth enables Abraham to conceptualize a new religion from the old ways of the agrarian fertility religion. From the power of the terebinth to structure

3   Bozorgi *et al.* 2013; Stewart 2014; Yaniv and Dudai 2014.
4   Genesis 2.7.
5   Avrahami 2012.
6   Berlin and Brettler 2004, p.91; Sarna 1989; Spero 2008.
7   Peachey 1995.
8   Beckmann 2009.
9   Beckmann 2009; Chadwick 1976; Melena 1974; Peachey 1995.

the consciousness of his passage as a dream, mythic, or visionary landscape,[10] Abraham appears in a state of altered consciousness that remarkably resembles the healing process achieved at ancient dream healing sanctuaries. We know, for example, that the famous healing sanctuary of Asklepeios at Epidauros also featured the fragrance of sacred pine, cedar, and olive scents that infused the dreams of the supplicants seeking dream healing. Similarly, the prophet Jeremiah uses balm—a resinous exude from terebinth—as an image of spiritual healing:[11] "Is there no balm in Gilead? Can no physician be found? Why has healing not come to My poor people?[12] Howl over her! Get balm for her wounds: perhaps she can be healed."[13]

DREAMS AND DIVINITIES

While Abraham, recently circumcised at his new God's command, sits under the terebinth tree, extraordinary manifestations appear before him:

> The Lord appeared to him by the terebinths of Mamre; he was sitting at the entrance of the tent as the day grew hot. Looking up, he saw three men standing near him. As soon as he saw them, he ran from the entrance of the tent to greet them, bowing to the ground, he said, "My lords, if it please you, do not go on past your servant. Let a little water be brought, bathe your feet and recline under the tree..."[14]

....

10 Spero 2008.
11 Jeremiah 8.22; Cheshire 2003.
12 See Genesis 37.25; Jeremiah 15.18.
13 Jeremiah 51.8.
14 Genesis 18.1.

Here Abraham sits on the threshold, the symbolic liminal space that rests between the tent within and the landscape beyond—between, we shall see, his present and his past, and between dream and reality.[15] It is the place, designated with terebinths, where archetypal events occur (with Jacob, David and Goliath, Abimelech, Absalom, Joshua, etc.). At that median place, under the fragrant terebinth tree, Abraham's drama unfolds.

Abraham sits under the terebinth tree "as the day grew hot." Terebinth, as a volatile essential oil, is strongest when the ambient heat is intense. Abraham relies on the cognitive enhancement that terebinth offers as he makes his way into a new paradigm of religious belief. Certainly, his new god has promised him much—abundant wealth, limitless progeny, superior force—but can Abraham trust these new visions as authentic and truthful, and as consistent with his own conscience and beliefs, or are they simply the hallucinations of a new god with the same excesses of ancient fertility rites and child sacrifice? These are the rituals held under the terebinth trees against which the Prophets continually rile. "You will be ashamed," warns Isaiah,[16] "Because of the terebinths that you have desired." Other atrocities are also cited as part of these practices:

> You who inflame yourselves [in frenzied idolatrous rites]
> Among the terebinths,
> Under every verdant tree;
> Who slaughter children in the wadis...[17]

....

15   Winnicott 1971.
16   Isaiah 1.29.
17   Isaiah 57.5 (see Deuteronomy 12.2; Jeremiah 2.20; Hosea 4.13).

Choosing to build his altars and to call on his god under the same terebinth trees, how can Abraham be confident that he is not deceived by these other powers? This is the core dilemma that Abraham must resolve. At a later time, Jacob seeks to commune with God and is instructed to bury his foreign idols under the terebinth and purify himself before approaching God through dream.[18] Abraham has chosen to defy the religious status quo by establishing his altars under the same terebinth trees. Abraham, I will show, challenges old beliefs in the making of his new god by using the same religious framework with new content.

The agricultural context of Abraham's new religion is often overlooked as his adventures are interpreted from the distance of contemporary concerns. From Kirkegaard to Lacan, and many in between, writers use the story of the near-sacrifice of Isaac—the binding or Akedah—as a projection screen for current existential concerns from Protestantism to Postmodernism.[19] But, do we recognize those concerns as the same issues that would have troubled a second millennium biblical patriarch? It seems unlikely.

Abraham comes from an agrarian social structure and seeks to devise his new religion from that context. Thus, the dimensions, values, practices, and themes of agrarian religion are immediately relevant to the background and future of Abraham's new religion. In this way, we may see how and when he uses its dimensions in the formulation of his new system of belief, and how and when he diverges from that belief system. For example, Abraham's construction of altars under the sacred terebinth trees traces back to ancient tree worship and agrarian fertility rites practiced under

18 Genesis 35.4, 35.8.
19 Abram 2003; Beach and Powell 2014.

those trees. Necessarily, Abraham uses the same context to express, define, and normalize his new vision, as that is the belief system against which he practices his new faith. When he "calls on the Name of God" under the tree, he demonstrates the pre-Mosaic religion that he holds. In other words, Abraham is claiming his god as primary among many gods that characterize agrarian Canaanite religion. It is not until Moses that the singularity of the ancient Israelite god is proclaimed. In that form, the planting of trees within an altar area was specifically prohibited.[20]

Similarly, we must analyze other components of this narrative in the context of ancient agrarian rituals and practices. The three visitors that Abraham receives under the terebinth tree correspond to cycles and structures of myths of oral cultures of this period.[21] Three otherworldly visitors typically present the hero with three challenges that he must conquer to demonstrate his authentic heroism. Hereby, we may interpret the three divine strangers as dream apparitions that present Abraham with his conscious-state conundrums to resolve. A divine form appears in each of Abraham's challenges: at Sodom, to announce Sarah's pregnancy, and to rescue Isaac from the sacrificial knife. These are not God's tests of Abraham as is often proposed, but, we will see, they are Abraham's questions in his terebinth dream state—Abraham's tests of God—concerning the veracity of his new reality and religion.

Islamic versions of this story highlight the dream message that Abraham received. Questioning the dream's veracity is fundamental to the telling of this tale. In this version of the story, Abraham is told to sacrifice his son, which, in Islamic tradition, is interpreted to mean his first-born son Ishmael,

----

20 Deuteronomy 16.21; Berlin and Brettler 2004, p.91.
21 Eliade 1957.

child of Sarah's handmaid, Hagar.[22] And there are other differences. Here, Abraham is not commanded by God to sacrifice his son. Instead, the command appears to Abraham in a dream. The divine voice instructs him accordingly:

> We immediately removed this thought from Abraham's mind and called out to him, "O Abraham, You considered your dream as Allah's command and laid your son for the purposes of slaughtering him! This was not Our command, but merely a dream of yours. Therefore, we have saved you and your son from this. We have done so because We keep those who lead their lives according to Divine guidance safe from such mishaps."[23]

DIVINE LAUGHTER

In local worship, Israelite women worshiped the "queen of Heaven" (Asherah) as the source of fertility. Archaeological evidence shows that jugs of terebinth were dedicated to this native goddess.[24] To make sense of his new vision, Abraham must employ the familiar framework of agrarian myth and ritual. At the same time, he must distinguish his vision from its preceding context of meaning. This mismatched overlay is most aptly witnessed in the announcement of Sarah's pregnancy. How can Sarah, an infertile wife, compete with the fertility goddesses of pre-Israelite religion? Sarah must usurp the identity of the local goddess, Asherah, the tree goddess and Queen of Sacred Groves and Terebinth Trees, to define a new religious order. In this way, God's announcement

....

22 Sura 37.100–111.
23 Sura 37.104–105.
24 King and Stager 2001.

of Sarah's imminent pregnancy is re-enactment of the "sacred marriage" of agrarian mythology and ritual.[25] It demonstrates the fertility of the new reality that can triumph over and against the old ways. After all, didn't God promise Abraham progeny greater in number than the stars of the heaven and sands of the sea?

Sarah herself is surprised by this tactic:

> And Sarah laughed to herself, saying, "Now that I am withered, am I to have enjoyment—with my husband so old?" Then the Lord said to Abraham, "Why did Sarah laugh...?" ... Sarah lied, saying "I did not laugh," for she was frightened. But He replied, "You did laugh."[26]

Sarah's laughter at God's announcement is a familiar symbolic referent to impregnation; it represents a release of repressed resistances that impede fecundity and prohibit the life-fulfilling force to manifest itself.[27] The ancient Greek goddess of agriculture, Demeter, laughs similarly. Angry over the loss of her daughter, she prohibits agriculture, risking the existences of both gods and men. When a bawdy dwarf named Baubo performs an obscene dance before her, Demeter laughs over the sight of a child in Baubo's womb; reconciliation is secured and agriculture is renewed.[28]

The passage announcing Sarah's god-given fertility is filled with laughter. The emphasis is on the breath. Abraham, Sarah, Sarah's community, even baby Ismael (using a pun on Isaac's name), though he quickly gets slapped down, and,

---

25 Gilhus 1997.
26 Genesis 18.12–15.
27 Barron 1999; Berger 1997; Raj and Dempsey 2010.
28 Devereux 1983.

later, Isaac, too, is laughing.[29] Laughter and play is the sign of a transitional space, a domain where tension is cleared, repression is released, and identity is reconfigured.[30] Whereas the Sodom episode was Abraham's attempt to redefine the divine as just and compassionate, Sarah's episode is a focus on psychological and spiritual change and growth. Laughter is the psychological mood of transitional space as it challenges established rules and authority to enlarge and enhance consciousness. Laughing, Sarah achieves a new status as wife and mother, and authority as matriarch.

If we consider the text itself as transitional, then we must examine the power of its words to indicate that alternative spiritual reality. Philo, the Hellenistic Jewish writer, did exactly that to explain Sarah's pregnancy as an act—both spiritual and physical—that reveals her union with God.[31] In transitional space, meaning is necessarily coded and left to the reader and audience to decipher. Whereas we examined this meaning through study of the aromatic aspect of sacred trees and ancient tree worship, Philo is explicit that Sarah experienced a mystical union with the divine.[32] He decodes this passage by interpreting the role of laughter in the transitional space of mystical experience.

According to Philo, it is God who is the father of Isaac, and he uses the text as evidence. Since Isaac, whose name means "laughter," is said by Sarah that "God has caused me laughter,"[33] Philo concludes that Isaac is the god-given force of joy in the universe. Thereby, he interprets Sarah's

---

29 See Genesis 17.17, 18.12, 15, 21.6, 21.9, 26.8.
30 Winnicott 1971.
31 Goodenough 1935.
32 Goodenough 1935; Yonge 2013.
33 Genesis 21.6.

pregnancy as a union of mystical significance that infuses the world with consciousness. In this version, "Philo insists that Isaac was not born a man, but as a pure thought."[34] Isaac, the joyful one, is the divine power of God's power of "sowing and begetting happiness in the soul." This episode, then, is a sacred marriage of agrarian rites. Terebinth, as cosmic tree, provides the passageway.

JUST IN TIME

Scholars have noted Abraham's willing acceptance of God's order to sacrifice Isaac as contradictory with his previous vociferous defense of the citizens of Sodom. However, this seeming inconsistency is eminently logical in the ways of dreaming. There, what is transgressive during the day and forbidden in waking thought, emerges for expression in the symbolic landscapes of nocturnal visions. Abraham reverses the roles of actor and the action as his method of releasing repressed thoughts and emotions. That is, it is not God who is testing Abraham, but Abraham who is testing his new god through the reversals of dream language, processing, and imagery. In this cognitive landscape, Abraham questions his god. Will he accept the sacrifice and confirm the old practices, or will he forge a testament of truth as promised under the terebinth tree of teaching?

When Abraham answers Isaac with the enigmatic words "God will provide,"[35] his response makes sense from the perspective of Abraham's religious re-envisioning and questioning of the true identity of his new god. With this

....
34 Schwartz 2004, p.336.
35 Genesis 22.14.

phrase, Abraham demonstrates his faith in his new deity to be the god that he envisions. His dream confidence overcomes his willingness to re-enact that very agrarian ritual of child sacrifice that he rejects. If his god is true, Abraham's god will provide the sacrificial victim to replace the sacrilege of child sacrifice. If his god is unfaithful, his son, too, is a scam and hallucination of religious and mental delusion. Abraham tests God in such a dramatic manner by enacting the very sacrifice that is offered to fill the demanding deity of agrarian child sacrifice. Will he accept it? He *must* "provide."

How could it be otherwise? If God is testing Abraham, why would he demand Abraham to perform an agrarian fertility rite? However, if Abraham is testing the identity of the divine voice that he hears under the fragrant terebinth tree and the true nature of his religious experience, then his faith is demonstrated in the words "God will provide." To sacrifice a child is the very definition of idolatry, not divinity, explains the prophet Jeremiah quoting God: "And they have built the shrines...to burn their sons and daughters in the fire—which I never commanded, which never came to My mind."[36]

This is a terebinth test and one of his three otherworldly terebinth guests will appear to confirm this tripartite challenge. The third angel of the three that appeared to Abraham under the terebinth tree, that original place of teaching and learning, will reappear here at the Akedah. Consistent with the visionary experience of terebinth, Abraham names this site accordingly as the place of divine encounter: "And Abraham named that site Adonai-*yireh*, whence the present saying, 'On the mount of the Lord there is vision.'"[37]

---

36 Jeremiah 7.31.
37 Genesis 22.14.

CONCLUSION

This mythic framework for the holiness of fragrant trees carries into later Jewish beliefs and survives today. From Greece to Cyprus to Gilead, votive rags are hung on terebinth trees as prayers for healing.[38] Scent is life itself and, as breath, creates the world.[39] Fragrant trees, specifically the terebinth, mark the primordial place of original creation. The scented tree facilitates travel between realms.

In folk beliefs, Abraham's terebinth tree is believed to be a manifestation of the sacred tree of Paradise.[40] It is humanity's attempt, our second chance, to restore original unity. Abraham appears here as healer, planting terebinths at each settlement he establishes. They contain curative powers with existential potencies. The terebinths he plants represent a testament to the healing of humanity. Thus, terebinth promises more than simply providing physical healing properties; it promises access to divine realms of curative consciousness. By using this focus on this essential oil, we are given a unique understanding of the religious significance of these biblical passages and of the possibilities and varieties of human spiritual experience and expression.

BIBLIOGRAPHY

Abram, D. (2003) "The Suffering of a Single Child: Uses of an Image from the Holocaust." Unpublished doctoral dissertation. Harvard University Graduate School of Education.

Avrahami, Y. (2012) *The Senses of the Scripture: Sensory Perception in the Hebrew Bible*. New York: Bloomsbury.

---

38 Hageneder 2005; Musselman 2002.
39 Genesis 2.7.
40 Schwartz 2004.

Barron, J. (ed.) (1999) *Humor and Psyche: Psychoanalytic Perspectives*. New York: Routledge.

Beach, B. and Powell, M. (eds) (2014) *Interpreting Abraham: Journeys to Moriah*. Minneapolis, MN: Fortress Press.

Beckmann, S. (2009) "Resin and Ritual Purification: Terebinth in Eastern Mediterranean Bronze Age Cult." Athanasia International Archaeological Conference, Rhodes, Greece.

Berger, P. (1997) *Redeeming Laughter: The Comic Dimension of Human Experience*. Berlin: Walter de Gruyter.

Berlin, A. and Brettler, M.Z. (eds) (2004) *The Jewish Study Bible*. New York: Oxford University Press.

Bozorgi, M., Memariani, Z., Mobil, M., Salehi Surmaghi, M.H., Shams-Ardekani, M.R., and Rahimi, R. (2013) "Five Pistacia species (P. vera, P. atlantica, P. terebinthus, P. khinjuk, and P. lentiscus): A review of their traditional uses, phytochemistry, and pharmacology." *Scientific World Journal*, doi: 10.1155/2013/219815.

Chadwick, J. (1976) *The Mycenaean World*. Cambridge: Cambridge University Press.

Cheshire, W. (2003) "Twigs of terebinth: the ethical origins of the hospital in the Judaeo-Christian tradition." *Ethics & Medicine 19*, 3, 143.

Devereux, G. (1983) *Baubo La Vulve Mythique*. Paris: Jean-Cyrille Godefroy.

Eliade, M. (1957) *Myths, Dreams, and Mysteries: An Encounter between Contemporary Faith an Archaic Realities*. New York: Harper Torchbooks.

Gilhus, I.S. (1997) *Laughing Gods, Weeping Virgins: Laughter in the History of Religion*. New York: Routledge.

Goodenough, E. (1935) *By Light, Light: The Mystic Gospel of Hellenistic Judaism*. New Haven: Oxford University Press.

Hageneder, F. (2005) *The Meaning of Trees*. San Francisco, CA: Chronicle Books.

King, P. and Stager, L. (2001) *Life in Biblical Israel*. Louisville, KY: WJK Press.

McClintock, J. and Strong, J. (1981) *Cyclopedia of Biblical, Theological, and Ecclesiastical Literature*. Grand Rapids, MI: Baker Book House (reprint of Harper and Brothers, 1867–1887).

Melena, J. (1974) "Ki-ta-no en las tablillas de Cnoso." *Durius 2*, 45–55.

Musselman, L.J. (2002) *Figs, Dates, Laurel, and Myrrh: Plants of the Bible and Quran*. Portland, OR: Timber Press.

Peachey, C.P. (May 1995) "Terebinth Resin in Antiquity: Possible Uses in the Late Bronze Age Aegean Religion." Master of Arts thesis, Texas A&M University.

Raj, S. and Dempsey, C. (eds) (2010) *Sacred Play: Ritual Levity and Humor in South Asian Religions*. New York: SUNY Press.

Sarna, N. (1989) *The JPS Torah Commentary Genesis*. Philadelphia, PA: The Jewish Publication Society.

Schwartz, H. (2004) *Tree of Souls: The Mythology of Judaism*. New York: Oxford University Press.

Spero, S. (2008) "But Abraham stood yet before the Lord." *Jewish Bible Quarterly 36*, 1.

Stewart, D. (2014) *Healing Oils of the Bible*. Marble Hill, MO: Care Publications.

Winnicott, D.W. (1971) *Playing and Reality*. London: Tavistock Publications.

Yaniv, Z. and Dudai, N. (eds) (2014) *Medicinal and Aromatic Plants of the Middle-East*. Heidelberg: Dordrecht Springer Science+Business Media.

Yonge, C.D. (trans.) (2013) *The Works of Philo*. Peabody, MA: Hendrickson Publishers.

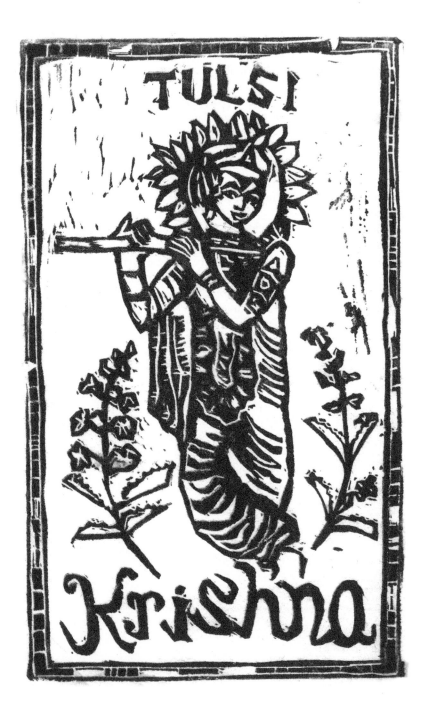

CHAPTER 5

CREATING PRESENCE

Holy Basil (Tulsi) and Hindu Devotional Performance

INTRODUCTION

Tulsi (*Ocimum sanctum*) extends this study with an opportunity to examine a ritual whose intent is to create an altered state of being in its devotees. The fragrant tulsi plant is the focus of an annual Hindu women's ritual that brings about an integrated consciousness through physical and ritual acts of worship. The versatility and effectiveness of tulsi to treat a wide variety of mental and physical ailments and illnesses makes this plant one of the holiest—and most useful—of the Indian pharmacological repertoire. It also presents a metaphorical model for cognitive unity, or, in religious terms, for union with the divine. In this state of mind duality is reconstructed into a powerful sense of unity and union, articulated as an encounter with the divine bridegroom, Krishna.

Apart from the lotus flower, sacred basil (tulsi) is the most holy plant in the Indian repertoire of plants and perhaps the most powerful herb for treating a range of physical and psychological concerns. "Nothing," the popular expression asserts, "equals the virtues of tulsi" (*tulasi tulana ateva tulasi*). From the common cold to cancer treatments, tulsi (*Ocimum sanctum*) has been described as "an herb for all reasons."[1] Significant to this study is tulsi's effect on the mind. Its potency has been equated with diazapam and anti-depressant drugs and its beneficial effect on memory and cognitive functioning is well documented. These properties complement the spiritual practices with tulsi that focus on mind and emotion and facilitate their integration. In this study, we witness tulsi's biological effects to reinforce the cultural narrative that employs tulsi imagery, tulsi metaphors, tulsi practices, and tulsi mythology. This Vaishnavite religious tradition articulates this higher level of consciousness and its acquisition.

Tulsi is the herb of transcendence.[2] It is sacred to the Hindu god Vishnu, worshiped with ornamental offerings of tulsi garlands by his devotees (named after him as Vaishnavites). Preeminent scholar of the anthropology of scent James McHugh rightly claims that, in academic inquiry, we currently have no scale or model to categorize scents. He explains that "the nature and significance of ornamentation with aromatic materials remains largely unexplored."[3] This is not the case with the Vaishnavites. Their writings—devotional poetry—use the landscape and flowers as codes for human emotions.[4] For the Vaishnavites, the scents emitted from plants are rich sources of meaning. Tulsi, in particular, conveys transcendent significance.

1 Cohen 2014, p.251; Mondal, Mirdha, and Mahapatra 2009.
2 Shrimad Bhagavatam 3.15.19; Krishna and Amirthalingam 2014.
3 McHugh 2011, p.157; 2012.
4 Dehejia 1990, p.23; Hardy 1983; Shuddhatmamata 2010; Venkatesan 2010.

THE SENSE OF SCENTS

Using jasmine as her example, scholar of Hindu religion Prataraji Shuddhatmamata explains this system, in which "Jasmine is both a flower as well as a mood."[5] For example, in a Vaishnavite maiden ritual called *pavai*, "the vow," during which the girls wait for their divine bridegroom to appear, the scent of jasmine anticipates the imminent arrival of the divine presence. Since jasmine blooms during the long monsoon season, it represents "the lover's mood of patient waiting for the absent one...associated with the rainy season, for the jasmine bloom most profusely then."[6] Elsewhere the Vaishvanite Alvar poet-saint Antal describes the pervasive sensuality of the awakening that jasmine represents, "the eastern wind blows softly over *mullai* [jasmine] wafting their fragrance everywhere."[7]

The tulsi ritual I examine in this chapter is performed by young women in their devotional and communal worship of the god Vishnu (Krishna). Called Vaishnava, this Hindu sect honors the poetic verses of their Alvar saints as sacred texts. Beyond the beauty of the poetry that provides the evidence for my study of holy basil and enhanced consciousness, these writings were intended to promote the unity of the devotee with her god, represented as the "divine bridegroom" in the poems. It is the mystical union that produces integration of mind, emotion, spirit, and body. The female Vaishvanite saint Antal achieved status as goddess through her experience with tulsi and her story is the model that the girl devotees assume in their performance of the *pavai* rite.

....

5   Shuddhatmamata 2010, pp.3, 31.

6   Shuddhatmamata 2010, pp.3-4.

7   Shuddhatmamata 2010, p.91.

Differentiating similar emotional states through a variety of fragrant flowers serves to describe the dimensions of the experience of divine union and unified consciousness. It also serves to focus the devotee on the intensity of that experience of separation. Separation provides the initial focus of the maidens' rite as they move, through the structure of the ritual performance, to welcome the presence of the divine. The rite is constructed through scent, space, and narrative to create that outcome of unified consciousness. Rather than alienate the worshiper through this initial concentration on separation, the constant focus on *absence*, contrariwise, serves to emphasize and anticipate the coming *presence* of the missing beloved. For example, when Antal's poem's *pavai* maidens wonder about the lingering scent of tulsi, they assume that it testifies to the fact that Krishna has visited recently.[8] The ultimate sign of that divine presence is the scent of tulsi.

The particular spiritual code for the mystical tulsi plant has a unique meaning in the sacred texts of the Vishnavite tradition written by the Alvar poet saints. Tulsi appears in many of Antal's verses and in Alvarite poetry in general where we see tulsi as representing the presence of the divine and, I propose, also its absence, joined in mystical unity. To put this in psychological terms, we are looking to replace cognitive dissonance (the absence or separation) with unified consciousness (the presence or integration). The use of tulsi points to a paradoxical understanding that puts absence and presence together. In contrast, *lack of fragrance* signals a state of being *devoid* of the divine, but the absence emphasizes its imminent presence. We see that fundamental unity in the maiden yearning for the divine bridegroom in a verse by Antal:

8   Venkatesan 2010, p.103.

Bring me his sacred basil
Cool, lustrous, blue,
Place it upon my glossy hair[9]

The maiden in this verse does not yet have the ritual wreath, signaling her separation from the divine, but she describes the culmination of the rite when she will achieve union and wear the tulsi wreath.

The popular saying that tulsi is "the meeting point of heaven and earth"[10] reflects this paradox. The tulsi plant initially signals separation, as described in this verse from one of Antal's poems expressing her yearning for the beloved presence: "Madly raving the names of the tulsi-wearing Lord, my heart is set on him alone."[11] The pain of separation is deeply felt as she speaks in the voice of her companion who witnesses her suffering:

...sad indeed is your plight,
Your gentle soul stands withered;
burnt are you
By the desire to get
the tulsi garland cool and bright,
Worn by our Lord with large lotus-eyes
and lips of red hue"[12]

One of the most evocative images of the distance that separates the Lover and the Beloved is in the poem where the maiden begs the dragonfly "to go to her Lord and then return to her bearing the fragrance of His tulsi garland."[13] Later she

....

9   Dehejia 1990, p.35.
10 Dehejia 1990, p.35.
11 Gupta 2013, p.54.
12 Gupta 2013, p.36.
13 Venkatesan 2010, p.121.

laments: "He denies his Tulsi wreath to my asking-weeping-self..." to express the plight and pangs of her separation.

However, we must also remember that tulsi is a paradox, and so it must indicate union as well as separation. It signals the presence of the divine that is immediate and immanent. For example, consider this line in Antal's poetry that describes the divine bridegroom's hair as scented with tulsi:

> We praise Narayana [Vishnu/Krishna] whose dark curls
> are fragrant with tulsi[14]

Perhaps we might not recognize the divine presence implicit in this line, but the ancient commentators certainly did. The commentators claim its meaning is obvious; that is, the perception of scent necessarily indicates the presence of the divine. This is their argument for the immanence of the divine presence through the scent of tulsi:

> They [ancient commentators] suggest an ingenious answer [to explain this line]: that the fragrance of tulsi must still hang in the air, causing the girls to speculate that Krishna had visited the sleeping girl on the previous night. This then leads the gopis [maidens] to wonder how long the fragrance of the tulsi entwined in Krishna's hair actually lasts. Finally, the gopis conclude that *since the fragrance of tulsi is so heady, Krishna must still be inside...*[15]

The poem mentions the bride's hair as scented similarly.[16] Tulsi, hereby, is the scent of divine transcendence and, paradoxically, its immediacy as well.

....

14 Venkatesan 2010, p.60.
15 Venkatesan 2010, p.102; author's emphasis.
16 Venkatesan 2010, p.15.

TALES OF TULSI

The myth that grounds this narrative is recounted in the Vaisnavite sacred literature where Antal's identity is also explained. There, we are told of a gardener and weaver of holy tulsi wreaths who was childless. One day, as he was tending his tulsi bushes, he discovered a baby girl beneath a tulsi plant. The gardener adopted the child, named her Kotai (later she would be renamed Antal), and raised her as his own. As priest of Vishnu, the gardener draped the statue of Vishnu with pure and fresh tulsi garlands every day. Little did he know that his daughter Kotai was so in love with Vishnu that she tried on the garlands each morning as she played the role of bride to her beloved Vishnu/Krishna, thus polluting the sacred necklaces with human touch. The gardener was enraged when he discovered the crime and forbade his daughter to approach the shrine again. Vishnu, however, had fallen in love with Kotai—Vishnu asserted that the tulsi wreath was doubly blessed by carrying her scent as well[17]—and her name became Antal, meaning "she who ruled," having conquered Vishnu's heart.[18]

The central image and defining moment of the Alvar founding myth is the wearing of the tulsi garland by the tulsi maiden. There, her offense of wearing the bridal tulsi wreath is pardoned and even celebrated by the god Vishnu that she supposedly offended by polluting the pure garland. Vishnu insists that she has actually intensified the holiness of the tulsi wreath "by adding her own personal scent to the necklace." We might wonder if he is referring to her human

....

17 Dehejia 1990, p.8.
18 Dehejia 1990, p.5.

scent—which would be a polluting act—or if she has added her tulsi scent (her divine identity) as a girl who was born in the earth under a tulsi bush to a maker of tulsi wreaths who becomes the bride of the tulsi-wearing lord.

The latter makes sense of the ending of the myth. As Kotai prepares to marry Vishnu, she steps toward the statue of the god and, unexpected to all present, Kotai disappears into the holy image. This is the recorded account of her "death." After this, she is known as Antal and worshiped as a goddess. Clearly, if she is the avatar of tulsi, her scent merges into the tulsi-garlanded Vishnu image, just as the story described that she "added more fragrance to the tulsi wreath of Vishnu." The accompanying maiden ritual is a mimesis of the Antal myth. At the dawn ritual, the garland that the image of Antal had worn all night is carried in procession to Vishnu's shrine. The ceremony represents "a crucial point in the legendary story of Antal's bakti [devotion], her total rejection of human love, her longing for union with the lord, and the lord's ultimate acceptance of her as a special devotee and as his bride."[19] To become the divine bride, hereby, is the goal of the maiden rite.

THE BLESSINGS OF UNION

In today's age of instant gratification and easy entitlement, the possibility of dedicating oneself to an intense practice over time may seem unlikely. For example, scholar Tim Betts's prescription for bringing epilepsy under control through mind exercises and aromatic inhalation was difficult to accomplish by patients because of these personality traits.[20] In study after

....
19 Dehejia 1990, p.6.
20 Betts 2003.

study, we see that people would rather take a pill to ease their pain or dysfunction than to commit to a long-term program of meditation, yoga, or aromatherapy.

Examining the Hindu practices and rituals concerning holy basil, however, offers us a window into the promise that sustained practice bestows. Additionally, the medicinal properties of tulsi confirm this outcome.[21] The outcome is integrated consciousness—a needed antidote to the depleted awareness, dissatisfaction, and divided consciousness that attitudes such as instant gratification and easy entitlement instill. This is not to say that the reader should assume the Hindu worship lightly. Instead, this chapter is intended to encourage and promote the qualities and skills of dedication, focus, and perseverance through committed practice.

We must examine the quality of consciousness that the ritual seeks to structure for its relevance to our mindset today. If we assume that contemporary society has created a state of divided consciousness, the lessons we may gain from this ritual that produces unified, embedded, and embodied consciousness are immense. To heal the divided mind—the disconnection between our intentions and our actions—requires a model and method that produces that outcome. This ritual named *pavai*—the "vow"—presents one such model.[22] It requires dedication and discipline that is performed over time to produce its benefits. Because these are the very characteristics that our consumer society rejects, this study provides an alternative model of social, personal, emotional, and aromatic healing. The intent is to challenge

....

21 Betts and Jackson 1998; Bhattacharyya *et al.* 2008; Dokania, Kishore, and Sharma 2011; Giridharan *et al.* 2011; Joshi and Parle 2006; Moinuddin *et al.* 2011; Saxena *et al.* 2012.

22 McDaniel 2003.

the priorities of our consumer society in its claim that retail therapy is our cure-all, with discovering the divine within ourselves that offers true healing and inner strength. Divine presence, hereby, indicates cognitive unity. Likewise, its absence demonstrates the opposite, as Antal tells us, "my mind runs/hither and thither/seeking his beautiful garland/of sacred basil/alas! I cannot control it."[23] It is, the poet claims, the tulsi wreath that makes the difference, "...if they place around my neck/His garland of sacred basil/Cool and green/Then alone shall I revive."[24]

Antal narrates a multitude of blessings that such union offers, such as:

fearlessness[25]

> I yearn, I melt
> Yet he says not,
> "have no fear."
> If willingly,
> He give his garland,
> Of holy basil,
> Bring it,
> Place it upon my breast.

serenity[26]

> Those who repeat these verses
> will never drown
> in the sea of sorrow

---

23   Dehejia 1990, p.111.
24   Dehejia 1990, p.121.
25   Dehejia 1990, p.124.
26   Dehejia 1990, p.27.

and fulfilment[27]

> If we worship Narayana
> Whose hair is adorned
> With the fragrant holy basil
> that holy one
> Will grant our desires.

TRAINING FOR TRANSCENDENCE

With this extensive mythological, ritualistic, and sensory background, we can now see that tulsi was a religious sensibility and also a powerful means of heightening consciousness and perception of the presence of the divine. The Vaishvanites use the scent of tulsi exclusively in the contexts of rituals and worship of the separation and union with the divine bridegroom. In this way, in Western psychological terminology, tulsi is used to create a conditioning trigger to bring about a particular quality of transcendent consciousness. The ritual that enacts this mythic cycle is structured to produce that cognitive outcome. It is a "progressive mystic journey."[28]

The first verses of the poem that accompany this women's ritual narrate the physical and moral requirements of participation:

> All you people of this world,
> Consider the rituals of our *pavai*-vow:

> We sing the praises of the supreme one
> who rests silently
> upon the ocean of milk.

....

27 Dehejia 1990, p.48.
28 Dehejia 1990, p.33.

We eat no ghee and drink no milk
and daily, we bathe before the dawn.

Kohl does not darken eyes
and flowers do not adorn our hair.

We do nothing that is wrong
and speak nothing that is evil.

Instead, we give freely
and offer alms to those in need

We live joyously,
trusting that all this will liberate us.[29]

Through ritual, the body is being prepared for the ultimate change of consciousness at the culmination of the month-long practice. Throughout this month of ritual fasting, bathing, and reading and reciting the story of Antal and her Beloved, the girls are preparing for its finale: union with the divine lover. That happens through story, performance, scent, and space. The culmination describes the Lover being hidden behind bedroom doors and it is up to the girls to rouse him from his slumber. The moment arrives when the doors of the temple open, revealing the statue of Antal, wearing fragrant tulsi garlands. They approach the image of Antal and, just as the myth narrated, they remove Antal's floral garlands, doubly scented, to place on the neck of Vishnu. In this way, by enacting the central act of the myth, the devotee becomes the divine beloved. The purpose of this sacred poetry was to enable and produce this transcendent transformation.[30]

....

29 Venkatesan 2010, p.52.
30 Venkatesan 2010, p.41.

CONCLUSION

Through narrative and experiential preparation, the maidens have been "conditioned" to experience this sacred moment as a transformation of awareness and entry into transcendent consciousness. This enhanced awareness is effected through the narrative, spiritual, and intersensory potency of the scent of tulsi. The ecstatic experience of tulsi is conditioned on and through multiple levels of meaning: in sacred narrative, ritual performance, and scent associated with space. All contribute toward a singular experience of divinity. The sacred poetry that describes and structures this experience is beautiful as poetry, but its purpose is to promote this quality of experience of unified awakened awareness.

There is much to learn from this ancient and modern practice. It is relevant to aromatic healing today because the Vaishnavite narrative *absence* of tulsi necessarily creates a profound realization of the unseen *presence* of the divine. The Vaishnavites recognize the inherent sacredness of this important plant that is both the avatar of the god Vishnu and of his enlightened devotees. Through this study we may learn poetical and powerful centering beliefs to influence, and perhaps even to incorporate into, healing practices. The focus on presence or what we might call *focused awareness* through the use of fragrant plants is relevant to our understanding of being, relationship, and service today.

BIBLIOGRAPHY

Betts, T. (2003) "Use of aromatherapy (with or without hypnosis) in the treatment of intractable epilepsy—a two year follow-up study." *Seizure: European Journal of Epilepsy 12*, 8, 534-538.

Betts, T. and Jackson, V. (1998) "Aromatherapy and epilepsy." *Epilepsy News 6*, September.

Bhattacharyya, D., Sur, T.K., Jana, U., and Debnath, P.K. (2008) "Controlled programmed trial of *Ocimum sanctum* leaf on generalized anxiety disorders." *Nepal Medical College 10*, 176-179.

Cohen, M. (2014) "Tulsi—Ocimum sanctum: a herb for all seasons." *Journal of Ayurveda Integrative Medicine 5*, 4, 251-259.

Dehejia, V. (1990) *Antal and Her Path of Love Poems of a Woman Saint from South India*. Albany, NY: State University of New York Press.

Dokania, M., Kishore, K., and Sharma, P.K. (2011) "Effect of Ocimum sanctum extract on sodium nitrite-induced experimental amnesia in mice." *Thai Journal of Pharmaceutical Science 35*, 123-130.

Giridharan, V.V., Thandavarayan, R.A., Mani, V., Ashok Dundapa, T., Watanabe, K., and Konishi, T. (2011) "*Ocimum sanctum* Linn. leaf extracts inhibit acetylcholinesterase and improve cognition in rats with experimentally induced dementia." *Journal of Medicine and Food 14*, 912-919.

Gupta, S. (2013) *Plant Myths and Traditions in India*. New Delhi: Munshiram Manoharial Publishers.

Hardy, F. (1983) *Viraha-Bhakti: The Early History of Krisna Devotion in South India*. Oxford: Oxford University Press.

Joshi, H. and Parle, M. (2006) "Cholinergic basis of memory improving effect of *Ocimum tenuiflorum* linn." *Indian Journal of Pharmaceutical Science 68*, 3, 364-365.

Krishna, N. and Amirthalingam, M. (2014) *Sacred Plants of India*. New York: Penguin Books.

McDaniel, J. (2003) *Making Virtuous Daughters and Wives: An Introduction to Women's Brata Rituals in Bengali Folk Religion*. Albany, NY: State University of New York Press.

McHugh, J. (2011) "Seeing scents: methodological reflections on the intersensory perception of aromatics in South Asian religions." *History of Religions 51*, 2, 156-177.

McHugh, J. (2012) *Sandalwood and Carrion: Smell in Indian Religion and Culture*. Oxford: Oxford University Press.

Moinuddin, G., Devi, K., Hanumantharayashetty, S., and Khajuria, D. (2011) "Comparative pharmacological evaluation of *Ocimum sanctum* and imipramine for antidepressant activity." *Latin American Journal of Pharmacy 30*, 435-439.

Mondal, S., Mirdha, R., and Mahapatra, S.C. (2009) "The science behind sacredness of Tulsi (Ocimum sanctum Linn.)." *Indian Journal of Physiological Pharmacology 53*, 4, 291-306.

Saxena, R.C., Singh, R., Kumar, P., Singh Negi, M.P., *et al.* (2012) "Efficacy of an extract of *Ocimum tenuiflorum* (OciBest) in the management of general stress: a double-blind, placebo-controlled study." *Evidence Based Complementary and Alternative Medicine 2012*, 1-7.

Shuddhatmamata, P. (2010) *The Divine World of the Alvars Lives and Songs of the Vaishnava Saints of South India.* Kolkata: The Ramakrishna Mission Institute of Culture. (First published 2003.)

Subramaniahn, K. (trans.) (2012) *Shrimad Bhagavatam.* New Delhi: Bharatiya Vidya Bhavan.

Venkatesan, A. (2010) *The Secret Garland: Antal's Tiruppavai and Nacciyar Tirumoli.* Oxford: Oxford University Press.

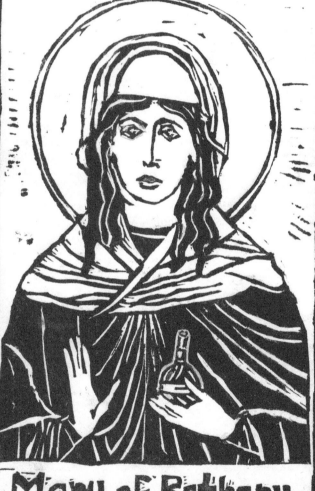

SPIKENARD

Mary of Bethany

CHAPTER 6

IN "MEMORY OF HER"

Healing with Spikenard in Biblical Times

INTRODUCTION

There's a passage in the gospel of John, when Martha tells her sister Mary that Jesus wants to talk with her, where the reader is presented with a conundrum. Translators of the text have questioned the meaning and intention of the adverb that Martha uses in this message. That adverb is *lathra* in Greek which translates literally as "secretly."

> When she [Martha] had said this, she went and called her sister Mary, saying *secretly*, "The teacher is here and is calling for you." And when she heard it, she rose quickly and went to him.[1]

Scholars attempt to make sense of this scene by translating *lathra* in such a way that it conveys their chosen narrative

....

1 John 11.28-29 (author's italics).

significance, which rests beyond the literal meaning of the word "secretly." Some translators replace *lathra* with the words "in private," others as "quietly," some as "whispering," and additional scholars employ other choices. None of these variants, however, are offered by New Testament Greek dictionaries as literal translations of this adverb.

The discrepancy between this word and its translations indicates a sensitive, fraught, and urgent moment in the narrative. Jesus had already spoken with Martha and had learned of her brother Lazarus's death when he informs Martha that he needs to speak with Mary—how? Alone? Secretly? Urgently? However one chooses to translate this adverb will demonstrate the interpretation one applies to this story.

For this chapter, I translate *lathra* not as "secretly" but as *privately*. We don't know what they talked about in private since, when we see the recorded conversation between Mary and Jesus, Mary simply repeats what Martha has already said openly to Jesus.[2]. I believe, however, that the effects of that private conversation become manifest, embodied, and enacted in Mary's demonstration of healing with Jesus—that is, her anointing of Jesus with the fragrant ointment of spikenard (*Nardostachys jatamansi,* also called *nard* in Greek):

It was Mary [of Bethany] who anointed the Lord with ointment and wiped his feet with her hair, whose brother Lazarus was ill.[3]

This descriptive verse is repeated and expanded in John 12.3:

---

2   John 11.21 and 32.
3   John 11.2.

Mary took a pound of costly ointment of pure [spike]nard and anointed the feet of Jesus and wiped his feet with her hair; and the house was filled with the fragrance of the ointment.

As German philosopher Gadamer explains, "all translation is interpretation."[4] The interpreter and what is interpreted necessarily merge to create a synthesis that speaks to the sensibilities and insights that the one offers the other. My aromatherapy perspective reveals the healing aspects of this narrative that are often ignored by other scholars who come with different biases and goals. A perspective is witnessed in the choice of translations that is offered at key moments in the text.

Using aromatherapy as an interpretive springboard offers an entry into an appreciation of the fragrant spikenard plant that also brings in cultural, literary, religious, and historical associations. It serves to contribute a more complex understanding than is possible without consideration of the details of the plant highlighted in the text. Jesus himself uses the pharmacological effect of spikenard—as sleep inducing—as a dominant spiritual and narrative metaphor in this gospel.

THE ALLIANCE OF JESUS AND MARY OF BETHANY

It is understandable that Mary seeks out Jesus for compassion and curing when her brother is deathly ill. Jesus had an affectionate relationship with the family, "and Jesus loved[5] Martha and her sister and Lazarus." The trust, intimacy, and

---

4   Gadamer 1975, p.384.
5   John 11.5: *eigapa*.

respect that Jesus and Mary share is palpable in these chapters. We witness their emotional mirroring of each other in Mary's grief over the loss of her brother Lazarus. Mary's weeping leads to Jesus's tears:

> Then Mary, when she came to where Jesus was and saw him, fell at his feet. When Jesus saw her weeping and the Jews who came with her also weeping, he was deeply moved in spirit and troubled...Jesus wept. So the Jews said, "See how he loved him [Lazarus]!" ... Then Jesus, deeply moved again, came to the tomb...[6]

That mutual admiration between Jesus and Mary was already evident when Jesus affirmed the superiority of Mary's contemplative mind as "the better way."

> Now they went on their way, he [Jesus] entered the village; and a woman named Martha received him into her house. And she had a sister called Mary, who sat at the Lord's feet and listened to his teaching. But Martha was distracted with much serving; and she went to him and said, "Lord, do you not care that my sister has left me to serve alone? Tell her then to help me." But the Lord answered her, "Martha, Martha, you are anxious and troubled by many things; one thing is needful. Mary has chosen the good portion, which shall not be taken away from her."[7]

Sitting at his feet and listening to his words, Mary demonstrates the embodied engagement that sets her apart—and at odds—with her active and goal-oriented sister Martha. This will be the thoughtfulness she employs to respond to the needs of Jesus through spikenard.

6   John 11.32–38.
7   Luke 10.38–42.

THE PSYCHOACTIVE EFFECTS
OF SPIKENARD

Currently designated as an endangered plant, spikenard grows in the Himalayas in Nepal, Tibet, Bhutan, and southwest China.[8] Export of the spikenard plant and parts is prohibited, but its essential oil is available for legal purchase. In biblical antiquity, the rhizome—the source of the most potent part of the plant—was one of the most prized and expensive fragrant plants, used in perfumes, incense, medicine, and ritual substances. The Gospel of John states that Mary had bought a highly refined product at the cost of 300 denarii for a Roman pound (327.45 grams or 11-12 ounces)—or an entire year's salary—so precious was this healing herb.[9]

Closely related to the psychoactive plant valerian, and effectively interchangeable for medical purposes, spikenard has a woody, floral, and slightly animalic scent. As an essential oil, spikenard is effective in producing a state of calm and relaxation, reducing anxiety, and treating insomnia. Spikenard works through two methods of application: inhalation and absorption. Its volatile oils affect the GABA receptors of the brain stem that control waking and sleeping.[10] By reducing the strength and duration of neuronal signaling, spikenard quiets the mind and relaxes the body. In addition to inhalation, another method of application of spikenard for sleep and relaxation is massaging the ointment or oil on the feet. Absorbed through the skin, spikenard—and its

8   Cropwatch; Gupta, Disket, and Mann 2012; M'Crindle 2005; Warmington 2014.
9   Levine and Brettler 2011, p.182, n.12.1-11.
10   Ito 2009; Mischoulon and Rosenbaum 2008; Takemoto *et al.* 2008; Takemoto *et al.* 2015; Takemoto, Yagura, and Ito 2009.

related valerian and lavender—produce deep relaxation and uninterrupted sleep (depending on the dosage).[11]

It is just what Jesus needs as the persecution and pursuit mount to his ultimate demise (fear of seizure and stoning[12]). Mary wisely selected this fragrant ointment for Jesus. Mary typically is given the epithet Myrrophore, the perfume (myrrh) carrier, for her use of plants in healing and burial. Here we see her expanded use of fragrant plants for psychological healing and religious faith.

The text does not directly describe Jesus falling asleep or feeling the effects of the application or inhalation of spikenard from Mary's activity. One line in the text, however, may have suggested exactly this outcome to an ancient audience: "The house was filled with the fragrance of the ointment."[13] Here, the *scent* of spikenard is highlighted. Relatedly, the ancient natural historian Pliny described the effect of breathing spikenard. He wrote that "the smell of [spikenard] induces sleep."[14] Thus, the scent of spikenard and its effect may be assumed to have been known by a general ancient audience. The text, hereby, implies that Mary has chosen this relaxing essential oil intentionally for this effect. Mary, in other words, has replicated the condition of consciousness that Jesus employed as a metaphor for death—sleep—it is the effect of the ointment. That is, when Jesus initially rejects the sisters' pleas to come and heal their ailing brother, Jesus dismisses their request with an alternative diagnosis of Lazarus's condition: "Our friend Lazarus has fallen asleep, but I go to awaken him out of sleep."[15] Simplemindedly, the disciples

11   Saeki 2000; Shen *et al.* 2005; Wormwood 2012.
12   John 11.8.
13   John 12.3.
14   Pliny 1940, p.21.
15   John 11.11.

take him literally, reminding Jesus that if Lazarus has only fallen asleep, "then he will recover."[16] Jesus, in an unusual act of direct speech, then "told them plainly, 'Lazarus is dead.'"[17]

In treating Jesus, Mary has given Jesus the respite and refuge that he so desperately needs. Why else would the authors of the books of Mark and Matthew claim that Mary—and Mary alone—is the single person to be mentioned each and every time the gospel is told throughout the world? Mary accomplished something crucially and substantively important. At a time of looming trauma, Mary offered healing consistent with Jesus's own narrative, that death is only a time of sleep from which to awaken.

METAPHORS, MOOD, AND MEANING

Clearly, Mary of Bethany chose spikenard specifically for its many levels of meaning: as precious oil, as a perfume, as a medicine, and as a display of faith, humility, love, and honor. Its psychoactive effects as a powerful sedative necessarily connect with Jesus's use of sleep as a metaphor for death. Importantly, we must recognize that Mary did not, in fact, actually *anoint* Jesus's feet in the sense of designating or foreshadowing his kingship. Instead, the text informs us that she "rubbed or massaged" (*eeleipsen*: literally, "smeared," from the verb *aleipho*) his feet with this potent oil. When she "wipes off" the ointment, a specific word is used that suggests "kneading" (*exemaksen*), suggesting again her healing activity. The act of anointing, usually applied to kingly or prophetic accession, carries religious significance while massaging is therapeutic. That word is used for the application of the oil on

16 John 11.12.
17 John 11.14.

the feet in both John and Luke. In the story in Matthew and Mark where the head is actually "anointed," the author uses the word "poured." Anointing the *feet* is not an act of kingly investiture.[18] What, then, is it?

Anointing is the word that is used when Jesus cures blindness by "anointing" (*epechrisen*)[19] the eyes of a blind man with clay and spittle in a previous chapter.[20] Here, however, Mary *massages* the feet of Jesus with the ointment. Jesus explains, quoting from Isaiah, that his power comes from above: "The spirit of the Lord is upon me because he has anointed me to bring good news to the poor."[21] As biblical scholar Teresa Hornsby explains, "*aleipho* describes the anointing of the sick. Anointing (*aleipho*) seems to signify good health and happiness, and its lack suggests sickness, sadness, and death."[22] Mary's gesture is an act of healing and of love, not of miraculous recovery and divine intervention as is Jesus's demonstration of curing represented through anointing. A skilled healer, Mary enacts the role of the loving disciple toward her Master. This explains why the scene with spikenard follows that enigmatic request of Mary by Jesus. With narrative logic, we may assume that the one is the outcome of the other—that is, Jesus's request to speak with Mary has something to do with her subsequent massage of his feet with spikenard.

In this example of sleep as death and death as sleep, Jesus establishes a basic spiritual metaphor that faith has the power to resurrect, just as a sleeping person may be awakened, as

....

18 Brown 1966; Carter and Levine 2013; Harvey 2006; Story 2009.
19 John 9.11.
20 John 9.3.
21 Luke 4.18.
22 Hornsby 2006, p.340.

he proclaims to Martha.[23] When we then witness Mary using a powerful sedative to massage Jesus's feet, she also is enacting this fundamental metaphor of faith that the sleeping (the dead) will awaken. Recognizing the inescapable death that Jesus will soon endure, awakening and resurrection (in the model of her brother Lazarus) is her urgent desire.

BEYOND BURIAL

Mary was treating Jesus with an aromatic sedative at the time of imminent death. It is exactly what Jesus, the man, requires during this heightened interlude of anxiety and mounting persecution. Because of these therapeutic properties of spikenard, we must consider Jesus's defense of Mary for her excessive use of precious spikenard. Jesus answers the disciples' charge by saying that Mary "has saved [*terese*: literally, "guarded"] the spikenard for my burial." Yet the narrative explains that, in fact, she has not saved it, but used its entire contents so that "the house was filled with fragrance of the ointment," provoking, also the disciples' charge of her wastefulness. Additionally, spikenard was not even used at traditional Jewish burials (as John 28 explains) and Mary, apart from Jesus's explanation to the disciples, did not attend the burial, according to John. We, then, may question Jesus's meaning with his statement that she guarded it for his burial.

Clement of Alexandria's oft-quoted line "too much perfume suggests a funeral" offers a clue about the metaphoric meaning of Mary's excessive application of spikenard and Jesus's enigmatic explanation. She has created the symbolic and physical context for Jesus to live out his narrative of sleep

---

23 John 11.25-27.

and death in this potent aromatic funereal setting. Jesus's use of the word for burial (*entaphiazein*) in fact suggests the preparation for burial, not the burial itself.[24] Just as Jesus insisted that Lazarus was in a condition of sleep in his death, Mary, likewise, has created the same narrative setting for Jesus. Her performance rests on the belief that resurrection from death is as predictable as waking from sleep. Accordingly, Mary is the first to visit and witness the empty burial vault after the crucifixion.[25]

Jesus's immediate concern is death, the harrowing and heartrending passage that he must make. It is the agony that we witness in his prayers in the Garden:

> "Father, if thou art willing, remove this cup from me; nevertheless not my will, but thine, be done." ... And being in an agony he prayed more earnestly; and his sweat became like great drops of blood falling down upon the ground.[26]

Ironically, in this hour of his *wakefulness* at Gethsemane, his disciples have fallen asleep beside him. Jesus relies on angelic presences to sustain him. Mary had given him a therapeutic, botanical, and spiritual model for this coming suffering to provide him with temporary respite by replicating the scents of sleep to tap into his spiritual sources of strength. Spikenard was the means of physical rest and affirmation of his spiritual narrative, that affirmation being tested later at the garden of Gethsemane.

To ignore the identity of the two—the psychoactivity of spikenard and Jesus's spiritual metaphor—is to neglect an

24 Varghese 2009, p.161.
25 John 20.
26 Luke 22.42-44.

important dimension of meaning in the text and an important method of healing in antiquity. By situating this study within the field of aromatherapy, we gain an important and otherwise irretrievable dimension of understanding. The beauty of the text, hereby, is amplified by this multidimensional study into the significance of spikenard in the Gospel of John.

CONCLUSION

Mary, as a skilled and sensitive aromatherapist, situates this act of healing—accomplished through the application of spikenard—within the narrative context that Jesus had already provided to his disciples, that death is simply a form of sleep, physically and spiritually. Mary, hereby, replicates Jesus's own spiritual metaphor to ease his anxiety and anticipation of actual death. By putting Jesus into a meditative and sedative state of mind, Mary provides an interlude of relief and relaxation for Jesus amidst the turmoil.

Mary's excessive application of spikenard fills the entire house with fragrance. Known for its sedative and soporific potencies, Mary effectively is treating Jesus's anxiety over his persecution and embodying his central metaphor of spiritual awakening from sleep. In this act of compassion, Mary reverses the role of caring for others that Jesus had always performed[27] to ministering to Jesus in his hour of need. Jesus and Mary had spoken "privately" because of the urgency of Jesus's last days and of the efficacy that the women disciples demonstrate (especially in comparison with the expressions of doubt and inattention displayed by the men). Mary wisely chooses spikenard to comfort Jesus in his state of persecution.

....

27 Mark 8.

She demonstrates her profound faith in him by sacrificing her family's wealth and her own feminine beauty to use her hair to wipe his feet. Mary, Jesus instructs, will be remembered because of her actions: "I [Jesus] tell you the truth, wherever this gospel is preached throughout the world, what she has done will also be told, in memory of her."[28]

This is the outcome of their private conversation.

BIBLIOGRAPHY

Brown, R. (1966) *The Gospel According to John*. Vol 1. Garden City, NY: Doubleday.

Carter, W. and Levine, A.-J. (eds) (2013) *The New Testament: Methods and Meanings*. Nashville, TN: Abingdon Press.

Cropwatch: www.cropwatch.org ("spikenard").

Gadamer, H.G. (1975) *Truth and Method*. New York: Seabury.

Giblin, C.H. (1992) "Mary's anointing for Jesus' burial-resurrection (John 12.1-8)." *Biblica 73*, 4, 560-564.

Gupta, R.K., Disket, J., and Mann, S. (2012) "A review on spikenard (nardostachysjatamansi DC.)—an 'endangered' essential herb of India." *International Journal of Pharmaceutical Chemistry 2*, 2, 52-60.

Harvey, S.A. (2006) *Scenting Salvation: Ancient Christianity and the Olfactory Imagination*. Berkeley, CA: University of California Press.

Hornsby, T. (2006) "Anointing Traditions." In A.-J. Levine, D.C. Allison, Jr., and J.D. Crosan (eds) *The Historical Jesus in Context*. Princeton, NJ: Princeton University Press, pp.339-342.

Ito, M. (2009) "Relaxing with fragrant vapor of natural medicine: its sedative effect on mice." *Aroma Research 10*, 3, 234-241.

Levine, A.-J., Allison, Jr., D.C., and Crosan, J.D. (eds) (2006) *The Historical Jesus in Context*. Princeton, NJ: Princeton University Press.

Levine, A.-J. and Brettler, M.Z. (2011) *The Jewish Annotated New Testament*. Oxford: Oxford University Press.

M'Crindle, J.W. (2005) *Ancient India as Described in Classical Literature*. Elibron Classics series. Westminster: Adamant Media Corp. Originally published 1901.

....

28 Matthew 26.13; Mark 14.9.

Mischoulon, D. and Rosenbaum, J.F. (2008) *Natural Medications for Psychiatric Disorders: Considering the Alternatives*. 2nd edition. New York and London: Lippincott Williams & Wilkins.

Pliny (1940) *Natural History*. Cambridge, MA: Harvard University Press.

Saeki, Y. (2000) "The effect of foot-bath with or without the essential oil of lavender on the autonomic nervous system: a randomized trial." *Complementary Therapies in Medicine 8*, 1, 2–7.

Shen, J., Niijima, A., Tanida, M., Horii, Y., Maeda, K., and Nagai, K. *et al.* (2005) "Olfactory stimulations with scent of lavender oil affects autonomus nerves, lipolysis, and appetite in rats." *Neuroscience Letters 383*, 1, 188–193.

Story, J.L. (2009) "Female and male in four anointing stories." *Priscilla Papers 23*, 4, 16–23.

Takemoto, H., Ito, M., Asada, Y., and Kobayashi, Y. (2015) "Inhalation administration of the sesquiterpenoid aristolen-1(10)-en-9-ol from Nardostachys chinensis has a sedative effect via the GABAergic system." *Planta Medica 81*, 5, 343–347.

Takemoto, H., Ito, M., Shiraki, T., Yagura, T., and Honda, G. (2008) "Sedative effects of vapor inhalation of agarwood oil and spikenard extract and identification of their active components." *Journal of Natural Medicines 62*, 1, 41–46.

Takemoto, H., Yagura, T., and Ito, M. (2009) "Evaluation of volatile components from spikenard: valerena-4,7(11)-diene is a highly active sedative compound." *Journal of Natural Medicines 63*, 4, 380–385.

Varghese, J. (2009) *The Imagery of Love in the Gospel of John*. Rome: Gregorian Biblical Press.

Warmington, E.H. (2014) *The Commerce between the Roman Empire and India*. Cambridge: Cambridge University Press. Originally published 1928.

Wormwood, V. (2012) *The Complete Book of Essential Oils & Aromatherapy*. Novato, CA: New World Library.

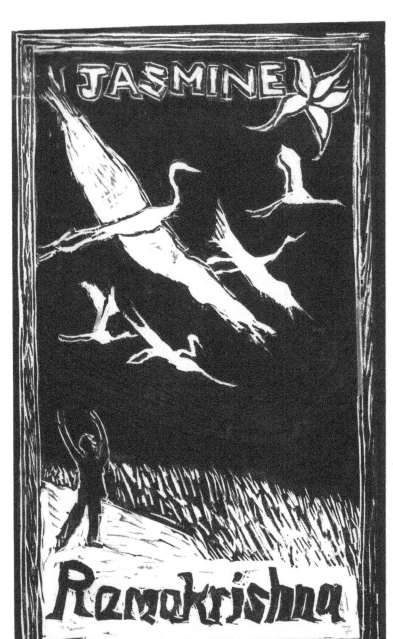

CHAPTER 7

THE SCENT OF JASMINE

Spanning the Divide between Epilepsy as Disability or as Extraordinary Experience through Cultural Context

INTRODUCTION

Jasmine (*Jasminum officinale*) continues the theme of the importance of studying the cultural context and personal life narrative for understanding construction of meaning. With a focus on the life of Sri Ramakrishna, we witness how biology may be interpreted differently depending on context. Culture has the power to change what the West might recognize as profound disability in need of medication to a demonstration of profound transcendence in a different cultural setting. Jasmine flowers, specifically, facilitate this transformation.

With the contemporary interest and prioritization of the brain for diagnostics, a new field named *neurotheology* has arisen.[1] This recent discipline seeks to trace the origin and impetus of experiences of altered consciousness as

---

1   Beauregard 2012; Miller 2013; Newberg 2010, 2012.

brain derived. Foremost in the controversy that this approach has aroused is the life of Sri Ramakrishna, the 19th-century mystic saint of Bengal, India. For his followers, Ramakrishna is an avatar of the divine in human form; his states of ecstasy are demonstration of his divinity, not evidence of his infirmity. For Western scientists, in contrast, Ramakrishna suffered from temporal lobe epilepsy that induced his states of loss of consciousness, dissociation, and seizure.[2]

This chapter makes no claim to resolving this controversy: neither am I claiming his divinity, nor, contrariwise, asserting his disability. Instead, I examine Ramakrishna's use of his human body to communicate his teachings and messages In either stance—as divine or mortal—Ramakrishna worked through his corporeal existence. From this perspective, we may see his physical symptoms as his means of achieving his spiritual reality. He worked in a specific cultural context that gave meaning to that expression. By examining Ramakrishna's mental state—epileptic or extraordinary—through the lens of culture, we may understand how this single condition of consciousness may be given divergent values, treatments, and outcomes.[3] Specifically, his use of jasmine flowers opens therapeutic pathways for aromatic healing today.

Even though all approaches identify the excitation of the brain as characteristic of epilepsy, each takes a different approach to its treatment. For standard "drug therapy.... Epilepsy is seen as an uncontrollable illness with unpredictable seizures, where medication is the only alternative."[4] Recent behavioral therapy has redefined epilepsy as a condition to be managed rather than a disease

....

2   Persinger 1983.
3   Turner *et al.* 1995.
4   Dahl and Lundgren 2008, p.248.

to be treated. Cognitive approaches control symptoms through mental strategies.[5] Similarly, Ayurvedic medicine recommends jasmine to treat physical and emotional imbalances.[6] Aromatherapy highlights the use of jasmine inhalation.[7] Cultural studies insist on the contextualization of any practice within its own cultural setting.[8]

EPILEPSY OR MEDITATING ON THE DIVINE?

Examining his initial experience of altered consciousness, we are told that Ramakrishna's symptoms were exacerbated by the recent death of his father and the stress of the strained financial circumstances that afflicted the family.[9] From this heightened emotional state, Ramakrishna experienced his first ecstasy at the age of six when he witnessed the flight of white cranes against a backdrop of black storm clouds.

> I was following a narrow path between the rice fields. I raised my eyes to the sky as I munched my rice. I saw a great black cloud spreading rapidly until it covered the heavens. Suddenly at the edge of cloud a flight of snow-white cranes passed over my head. The contrast was so beautiful that my spirit wandered far away. I lost consciousness and fell to the ground. The puffed rice was scattered. Somebody picked me up and carried me home

---

5   Dahl and Lundgren 2005.
6   Kapoor 2001.
7   Cooksley 2002; Life Science Publishing 2014; Mojay 1997.
8   Bhawuk 2003, 2011; Hofstede 1980; Kleinman 1981; Livermore 2013; Markus 1991; Misra, Srivastava, and Misra 2006; Wilce 2003; Wilce and Price 2003.
9   Nikhilananda 1953.

in his arms. An excess of joy and emotion overcame me...
This was the first time that I was seized with ecstasy.[10]

From a Western medical perspective, the resulting state of unconsciousness indicates a seizure characteristic of photosensitive (high contrast) epilepsy. In that state, the visual contrast of white and black will trigger an epileptic seizure.

However, from a traditional Hindu perspective, we are told that "his spirit wandered far away" and that Ramakrishna "meditated on the gods and goddesses"[11] as explanation of this interlude. It was an encounter with the divine world. This alternate explanation indicates a profound difference in perspective and attributed significance to the same episode, and, importantly, has immediate and tremendous consequences for behavior, available options, and beliefs concerning the nature of healing and reality.

The next time that we have evidence of a photosensitive trigger for Ramakrishna, we witness, again, an alternative attribution of meaning from a Western medical model of epilepsy. Then, Ramakrishna's wife, Sarada-devi, wove a thick seven-strand garland of jasmine flowers for the statue of the goddess Kali at her temple at Dakshineswar. She wrote of this incident:

> One day when visiting Dakshineswar, I made a big garland of seven strands with some jasmine and red flowers... I sent the garland to the Kali temple to adorn the image of Divine Mother. The ornaments were taken off from the body of Kali, and she was decorated with the garland. Sri Ramakrishna came to the temple. He at once fell into an ecstatic mood to see the beauty of Kali so much enhanced

10 Quoted in Rolland 2008, p.6.
11 Nikhilananda 1953.

by the flowers. Again and again, he said, "Ah, these flowers are so nicely set off against the dark complexion of the Divine Mother!..." I entered the temple and found Sri Ramakrishna singing, his voice trembling with love and devotion.[12]

In both of these examples of Ramakrishna's response to visual contrast, we see Ramakrishna excited by the beauty he witnessed that propels him into ecstasy.

"Jasmine is a flower as well as a mood," explains scholar of ancient Hindu religion, Pravrajika Shuddhatmamata.[13] In her work on the ecstatic religion of the south Indian Alvars, Shuddhatmamata explicates the symbols and codes of Hindu religious practice. The word "mood" (*bhava*) used here is not a simple or transitory emotional attitude, but an individual spiritual orientation and personal relationship with God. Different flowers indicate various ecstatic moods. Hence, jasmine signified "hopeful longing [for the divine]"[14] while the *neytal* flower refers to the subtly different sensibility of "anguished separation."[15] Both are examples of devotees' anticipation of ecstatic union with the divine bridegroom. Dedication of jasmine garlands brings great merit to the worshipers.[16] For Ramakrishna, Sarada-devi's jasmine garlands facilitated his union with the Goddess by inducing the ultimate ecstatic mood of *bhava-samadi* through his witness of divine beauty.

How we choose to understand this episode places us at an almost irreconcilable epistemological divide. Do we recognize

....

12   Nikhilananda 2004, p.78.
13   Shuddhatmamata 2003.
14   Shuddhatmamata 2003, pp.3, 31.
15   Shuddhatmamata 2003, p.4; Shuddhatmamata 2015.
16   Goody 1993.

Ramakrishna's response to the sight of the black and white image as medical epilepsy or as Hindu enlightenment? Or, is there a possibility to integrate both into a greater understanding of spirituality and the capacity of culture to redirect experience into frameworks of transcendent meaning rather than diagnoses of disability and illness? If we choose the Hindu pathway, what might that contribute to Western understanding and aromatherapeutic practice? From the viewpoint of aromatic healing, the answer is likely to rest in the fragrance of the flower, and, in this case, that flower is jasmine.

MEANS AND MEANING

Jasmine is used in aromatic healing as a method to treat epilepsy by inhaling this aromatic scent immediately before the attack, during the experience of the auras that commonly anticipate an epileptic seizure. Since 1881, doctors have known that an epileptic attack may be diverted through inhalation of a strong scent.[17] In aromatherapy, jasmine is the premiere scent for this purpose.[18]

Additionally, we must recognize that photosensitive epilepsy may be the cognitive pathway, but its significance and suffering (or lack thereof) is a cultural construct. We know, for example, that shamanistic religions oftentimes consider people with epilepsy to be specialists in spiritual domains.[19] Both ability and disability are defined by and experienced within the culture in which they are manifest. Thereby, we

....

17 Efron 1956.
18 Battaglia 2003; Life Science Publishing 2014; Richard and Reiter 1995.
19 Eliade 2004; Fadiman 1997; Kleinman 1981.

can only consider epilepsy as the neuronal *means* of achieving a certain state of consciousness, but not the *meaning* of that state of mind. Furthermore, even though we may recognize the similarities between a diagnosis of epilepsy and Ramakrishna's mood of bhava-samadhi, we cannot identify them as identical because of the stigma that is attached to mental conditions and illness in the Western world. "Not only does the world create a powerful negativity for those who suffer epilepsy, but it also projects a negative response on psychological well-being."[20] Ramakrishna's "mood" was a celebrated triumph in the religious and cultural contexts in which he lived and taught. Thus, even if the neuronal pathway is similar, their cultural expressions create vastly different conditions and states.

TREATING EPILEPSY WITH JASMINE

One of the most dramatic cases describing the use of jasmine to treat epilepsy is the 1956 story of a jazz singer. Her profound anxiety just before she was to perform on stage induced epileptic seizures.[21] Efron, working with this singer, prescribed jasmine inhalation to calm her. It worked.

German scientists recently hailed jasmine to be as powerfully effective as valium.[22] The authors of this study claim that their research "can be seen as evidence of the scientific basis for aromatherapy."[23] Jasmine acts on the brain's GABA receptors, which are responsible for the sleep/waking

....

20 Davidson n.d., p.1.
21 Efron 1956; Richard and Reiter 1995.
22 Sergeeva *et al.* 2010.
23 *Telegraph* 2010.

cycle and the neuronal excitability associated with epilepsy. Inhalation of jasmine moves the scent molecules from nose to lungs to blood to brain. It creates a "calming and hypnotic effect [that] depends solely on the dosage" thereby producing an effect as potent "as barbituates and propofol."[24] Similarly, anti-convulsive drugs that also interact with GABA receptors are used to treat epilepsy.[25]

In addition to stage performances, the jazz singer used jasmine for any situations likely to induce seizures and also at the start of seizures. Efron employed a conditioning program to teach the singer to interrupt the seizures: "When the singer had learned to successfully interrupt seizures using jasmine, Efron then conditioned the smell of jasmine to a bracelet, and finally to the thought of the bracelet." The study demonstrated that the singer was able to "counteract the increase in cortical activity associated with her seizure onset through conditioning...and it marked the beginning of conditioning as seizure therapy for patients with epilepsy."[26]

We recognize similar activity by Ramakrishna. According to Efron's method, the scent of jasmine should have averted the signal of the white on black as a photosensitive trigger. Instead, the statue of the black Kali decked with white jasmine flowers *triggered* Ramakrishna's bhava-samadi episode. In his own words, Ramakrishna's ecstasies were induced by the beauty he beheld before him. His excitation, which led to loss of consciousness, created an experience of awe and great pleasure. In various other episodes, Ramakrishna's

24 *Science Digest*, July 12, 2010.
25 NHS Choices, July 7, 2010.
26 Dahl and Lundgren 2008, pp.245-246.

capacity to induce, control, and enjoy these mental episodes demonstrates his agency over the process.

An example of Sri Ramakrishna's agency over mental states is shown in the following example. A potential devotee, Girish Ghosh, insists that he cannot maintain the spiritual practice that Sri Ramakrishna has recommended for him. Ramakrishna, in total control, offers to enter the state of enlightenment for Ghosh to witness, and he accomplishes that outcome on the spot:

> Alas, the Master was asking him to do such a simple thing and he was unable to agree to do it. Girish was in an embarrassing situation, but he remained calm and silent even though a tempest of anxiety, fear, and despondency was blowing in his mind. The Master looked at Girish again and said to him with a smile: "So you are unwilling to agree even to this. All right. Give me your [spiritual] power of attorney [to act on your behalf]." Immediately, the Master went into ecstasy![27]

This agency is affirmed by contemporary behavioral management techniques that use jasmine to control seizures. Neuroscientist Tim Betts has developed an effective cognitive-behavioral method that uses hypnosis (reinforced post-hypnotic suggestion to relax at the scent of jasmine oil) with jasmine that is reminiscent of the examples we have seen with Ramakrishna.[28] Ramakrishna demonstrated control over his flights into altered consciousness, just as jasmine and hypnosis enable people to control their symptoms today. Thus, we examine the behavioral training techniques used in the

----

27 Saradananda 2003, p.390.
28 Betts and Jackson 1998; Holmes, Schachter, and Kasteleijn-Nolst 2007.

jasmine-controlled epilepsy and discover similar structures and procedures that Ramakrishna necessarily employed as part of his priestly practice as a Hindu priest: daily collection and construction of fragrant floral garlands, breathing techniques (inhalation) in anticipation of meditation, and dietary regimens. With the cognitive approach, recent work by Dahl and Lundgren recommend secular versions of spiritual practices such as "acceptance, diffusion skills, mindfulness, and committed action."[29] Over time, such practice produces a more resilient brain and functioning.[30] Clearly, we cannot replicate the high cultural honor bestowed on those who attained control of conscious states and expressions of heightened spiritual experience and expression in India, but there is much to learn that can assist in aromatic healing with jasmine.

CONCLUSION

His culture offered Ramakrishna a deeper integration by contextualizing experience within a setting of divine devotion. His practice of religious worship, through fragrant flowers and meditation, gave him daily reinforcement and personal agency over variations in consciousness. While Western medical approaches to the treatment of epilepsy deny conscious control, and cognitive-behavioral techniques offer temporary effectiveness, spiritual practice, in an appropriate cultural setting, has the capacity and capability to transform a Western disability into experiences of extraordinary spiritual awareness.

....

29 Dahl and Lundgren 2008, p.252; see also Semple and Hatt 2012, pp.326–342.
30 Beauregard 2012; Miller 2013; Newberg 2010, 2012.

BIBLIOGRAPHY

Battaglia, S. (2003) *The Complete Guide to Aromatherapy*. Brisbane, Australia: The International Centre of Holistic Aromatherapy.

Beauregard, M. (2012) "Neuroimaging and Spiritual Practice." In L. Miller (ed.) *The Oxford Handbook of Psychology and Spirituality*. Oxford: Oxford University Press.

Betts, T. (2003) "Use of aromatherapy (with or without hypnosis) in the treatment of intractable epilepsy—a two year follow-up study." *Seizure: European Journal of Epilepsy 12*, 8, 534-538.

Betts, T. and Jackson. V. (1998) "Aromatherapy and Epilepsy." *Epilepsy News 6*.

Bhawuk, D. (2003) "Culture's influence on creativity: the case of Indian spirituality." *International Journal of Intercultural Relations 27*, 1-22.

Bhawuk, D. (2011) *Spirituality and Indian Psychology*. New York: Springer.

Cooksley, V. (2002) *Aromatherapy*. New York: Prentice Hall Press.

Dahl, J. and Lundgren, T. (2005) "Behavioral analysis of epilepsy: conditioning mechanisms, behavior technology, and the contribution of ACT." *The Behavioral Analyst Today 6*, 3, 191.

Dahl, J. and Lundgren, T. (2008) "Conditioning mechanisms, behavior technology, and contextual behavior therapy." *Neuropsychiatric and Behavioral Disorders* 245-252.

Davidson, Z. (n.d.) "Living with Epilepsy and Aromatic Oils." Available at theida.com/ew/wp/content/uploads/2010/10/1iving-with-epilepsy- and aromatic-oils.pdf, accessed on January 17, 2017.

Dehejia, V. (1990) *Antal and Her Path of Love*. Albany, NY: State University of New York Press.

Efron, R. (1956) "Effect of olfactory stimuli in arresting uncinate fits." *Brain 79*, 267-281.

Eliade, M. (2004) *Shamanism: Archaic Techniques of Ecstasy*. Princeton, NJ: Princeton University Press.

Fadiman, A. (1997) *The Spirit Catches You and You Fall Down: A Hmong Child, Her American Doctors, and the Collision of Two Cultures*. New York: Farrar, Strauss, and Giroux.

Goody, J. (1993) *The Culture of Flowers*. Cambridge: Cambridge University Press.

Hofstede, G. (1980) *Culture's Consequence: Comparing Values, Behaviors, Institutions, and Organizations across Nations*. Thousand Oaks, CA: Sage.

Holmes, G., Schachter, S., and Kasteleijn-Nolst, D. (2007) *Behavioral Aspects of Epilepsy: Principles and Practices*. New York: Demos Medical Publishing.

Kapoor, L.D. (2001) *Handbook of Ayurvedic Medicinal Plants*. New York: CRC Press.

Kleinman, A. (1981) *Patients and Healers in the Context of Culture: An Exploration of the Borderland between Anthropology, Medicine, and Psychiatry*. Berkeley, CA: University of California Press.

Life Science Publishing (2014) *Essential Oils Desk Reference*. Lehi, UT: Life Science.

Livermore, D. (2013) *Expand Your Borders*. Grand Rapids, MI: Baker Academic.

Markus, H. (1991) "Culture and the self: implications for cognition, emotion, and motivation." *Psychological Review 98*, 2, 224-253.

Miller, L. (ed.) (2013) *The Oxford Handbook of Psychology and Spirituality*. Oxford: Oxford University Press.

Misra, G., Srivastava, A., and Misra, I. (2006) "Culture and Facets of Creativity: The Indian Experience." In J. Kaufman and R. Sternberg (eds) *The International Handbook of Creativity*. Cambridge: Cambridge University Press, pp. 4421-456.

Mojay, G. (1997) *Aromatherapy for Healing the Spirit*. Rochester, VT: Healing Arts Press.

Newberg, A. (2010) *Principles of Neurotheology*. New York: Ashgate.

Newberg, A. (2012) "Transformation of Brain Structure and Spiritual Experience." In L. Miller (ed.) *The Oxford Handbook of Psychology and Spirituality*. Oxford: Oxford University Press.

NHS Choices (July 12, 2010) "Jasmine 'as Good as Valium' Claim." Available at www.nhs.uk/news/2010/July07/Pages/jasmine-for-anxiety.aspx, accessed on 17 January, 2017.

Nikhilananda (trans.) (2004) *Sri Sarada Devi, The Holy Mother: Her Teachings and Conversations*. Woodstock, VT: SkyLight Paths.

Nikhilananda (1953) *Vivekananda: A Biography*. New York: Ramakrishna-Vivekananda Center of New York (chapter: "At the Feet of Ramakrishna").

Persinger, M. (1983) "Religions and mystical experiences as artifacts of temporal lobe function: a general hypothesis." *Perceptual and Motor Skills 57*, 1255-1262.

Richard, A. and Reiter, J. (1995) *Epilepsy: A New Approach*. New York: Walker and Company.

Rolland, R. (2008) *The Life of Ramakrishna*. Kolkata: Advaita Ashrama.

Saradananda (2003) *Sri Ramakrishna and His Divine Play*. St Louis, MO: Vedanta Society of St. Louis.

Science Digest (July 9, 2010) "Intoxicating Fragrance: Jasmine as Valium Substitute."

Semple, R.J. and Hatt, S. (2012) "Translation of Eastern Meditative Disciplines into Western Psychotherapy." In L. Miller (ed.) *The Oxford Handbook of Psychology and Spirituality*. Oxford: Oxford University Press.

Sergeeva, O.A., Kletke, O., Kragler, A., Poppek, A., *et al.* (2010) "Fragrant dioxane derivatives identify beta1-subunit-containing GABAA receptors." *Journal of Biological Chemistry*. doi: 10.1074/jbc. M110.103309

Shuddhatmamata, P. (2003) *The Divine World of the Alvars Lives and Song of the Vaishnava Saints of South India*. Kolkata: The Ramakrishna Mission Institute of Culture.

Shuddhatmamata, P. (February 7, 2015) Personal communication.

Telegraph (July 10, 2010) "Smell of Jasmine as Calming as Valium."

Turner, R., Barnhous, R.T. Luckoff, D., and Lu, F.G. (1995) "Religious or spiritual problem? A culturally sensitive diagnostic category in the DSM-IV." *Journal of Nervous and Mental Disease 183*, 7, 435-444.

Wilce, J.M. (2003) *Social and Cultural Lives of Immune Systems*. New York: Routledge.

Wilce, J. and Price, L. (2003) "Metaphors our Bodyminds Live By." In J.M. Wilce (ed.) *Social and Cultural Lives of Immune Systems*. New York: Routledge.

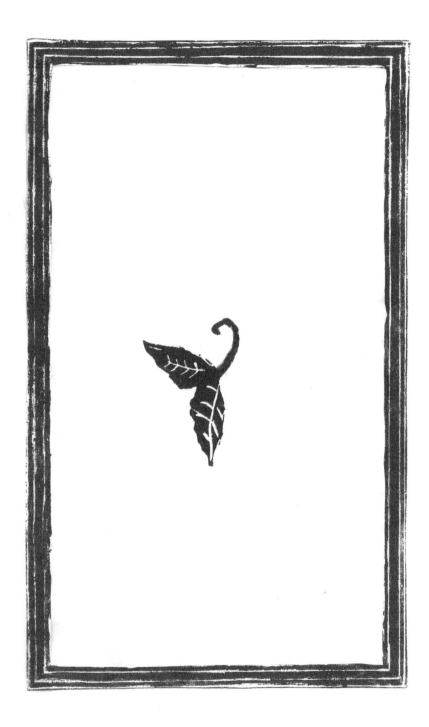

CONCLUSION

This book is my effort toward reclaiming the lost vitality of scent in our thoughts, lives, and relationships through stories of aromatic healing. This ability of scent to display its healing capacities is illustrated in the stories on aromatic olfaction that I consider in this collection. The human rejection of scent was a profound existential loss that left its mark in the human yearning for wholeness. Each vignette reveals this crisis and disruption in the narrative creation of self. The stories demonstrate the process of aromatic healing by revealing the divisions of self and showing the pathway to wholeness.

The divided self, what perfume scholar Stamelman identifies as an experience of "essence of absence"[1] at the core of the self, mirrors the processes of scent collection and perfume creation. He explains that the integration of an element of putrefaction or foul-smelling animalic substance (i.e., musk, civet, ambergris, castoreum) in the development of the most valuable perfumes provides a core symbolism of the aromatic imagination. Beauty is created out of dying flowers and rotted scents or what has been called "the foul and the fragrant" of the world of smell perception. There is

----

1   Stamelman 2006, p.19.

a basic paradox in their construction. This paradox asserts the existential realization that loss rests at the core of life, beauty, and sexuality.

The stories that I examine in this collection indicate that the realization of a paradoxical consciousness leads to an experience of human wholeness. The paradox must be confronted, embraced, and held in simultaneous legitimacy without too easily resolving either pole of the dichotomy. In these stories of the interactions of plants and people, it is scent that is the vehicle to achieve this integration. Set in diverse contexts of time and place, scent was accompanied by relevant cultural narratives that supply the missing links to greater understandings.

Sandalwood, in Chapter 1, demonstrates the power of narrative to construct reality. That construction, when situated within a meaningful cultural context, serves to prove the difference between living in a state of madness or discovering one's divinity and, thereby, becoming truly human. Through its psychoactive properties, the valued scent of sandalwood provided the means of healing, acting similarly to current anti-anxiety medications. Ramakrishna overcame madness to achieve divinity through this means.

In Chapter 2 on the *lotus*, I use the biblical narrative of Job as a model of the healing process through the metaphor of the journey and the challenges to consciousness that the journey holds. The adventures of Job and the lotus remind us that the outcome of suffering and healing is not an automatic success story, but is dependent on the realizations that accompany the healing process. What story is being told through suffering?

Job was able to travel a dark subterranean passage, represented by the scent of the narcotic blue water lily, and emerge into light. With its narcotic properties, the lotus (water lily) provides the psychoactive effect that matches the narrative of the underworld journey. Job secures an enhanced awareness through the confidence of his belief and his willingness to accept a larger frame of meaning of the divine than is comprehensible or comfortable to normal human consciousness. That is the goal of healing: an expanded consciousness. Thus, Job is an archetypal healer and the model of the shaman brought important aspects of aromatic healing to the foreground.

Focusing on the *neem* tree, Chapter 3 highlights a quality of paradoxical consciousness whereby opposites are united into a greater whole than is possible with only singular assumptions. This achievement is represented by the goddess Sitala Mata who both causes and cures disease, and who appears through the scent of neem in healing. I consider how her ancient rituals incorporates variolation (inoculation) that gave rise to this ambivalent identity whereby the disease and its cure arise from the same substance. For contemporary healing, the message of Sitala Mata's healing with neem is a greater acceptance of the complexity of living through welcoming former oppositions into a greater compassionate unity.

Chapter 4 on the fragrant *terebinth* tree examines a founding myth in the story of the biblical Abraham's establishment of a new monotheistic religion. Opening the breathing passageways and, thereby, expanding awareness, the scent of terebinth inspires Abraham's development of a fresh paradigm of faith and healing. It enables him to challenge systems of injustice and to formulate new models of belief.

The fragrant *tulsi* basil in Chapter 5 emphasizes the ritual performance of healing that necessitates dedication, persistence, and belief. Continuing the theme of paradoxical awareness as an expansion of consciousness, this chapter examines the poetry of the Hindu maiden's bridal ritual with the Lord Krishna. The experience of absence is complemented by the imminent presence of divine blessing that is heralded by the sweet scent of basil.

Chapter 6 on *spikenard*, a fragrant soporific plant, examines a well-known passage from the New Testament. It demonstrates how an aromatic analysis has the power to reveal deeper levels of meaning and emotion that were previously neglected in traditional scholarship. The scent of spikenard is a gift of healing, proving that scent, emotion, and meaning are companion sources of significance.

Chapter 7 on *jasmine* brings immediacy to this aromatherapeutic study through its examination of the use of jasmine in healing epilepsy today. The calming effects of the scent of jasmine offer a healing method that reinforces the agency and identity of individuals to create, control, and manage illness as a source of empowerment.

Each chapter contributes its own insight into the healing process. What they all share is the belief that healing is an inner phenomenon, not an external acquisition. Healing the body produces a simultaneous healing of mind, relationship, and community. Given the social history and hierarchy concerning the rejection of smell, especially in the West, the retrieval of smell as a vital sensory modality necessarily involves our societal practices and institutions as well.

My claim of the profound healing capacity of scent is a tall order for this single sensory modality. Yet, it is the direction to which the notion of paradoxical consciousness and integration leads us: to human wholeness through reclaiming scent and, thereby, enabling humans to achieve what it truly means to be "civilized."

BIBLIOGRAPHY

Stamelman, R. (2006) *Perfume: Joy, Obsession, Scandal, Sin.* New York: Rizzoli International Publications.

SELECTED SOURCES FOR ESSENTIAL OILS AND ABSOLUTES

Eden Botanicals
www.edenbotanicals.com
(707) 509-0041
(855) EDEN OIL

Liberty Natural Products
www.libertynatural.com
(800) 289-8427

Plant Therapy
www.planttherapy.com
(800) 917-6517

Stillpoint Aromatics
www.stillpointaromatics
(928) 301-8699

White Lotus Aromatics
www.whitelotusaromatics.com
(360) 457-9136

Whole Foods grocery stores also carry essential oils.

INDEX

Dorothy Abram (Ed.D. Harvard University) is a Professor of Psychology and Sociology at Johnson and Wales University. She applies her expertise and extensive explorations of the senses and sensuality, theater and the dramatic, morality and meaning, to the world of aromatherapy. Here you will discover totally fresh insights into the synergy of scent and the forces of life that captivate, culture and drive humans to great heights of ecstasy and excellence. Abram takes a close, detailed look at the role specific scents have had on the lives of major figures. Taking us on this journey Abram allows us to participate in the transformative effect of scent on the lives of others and hopefully on ourselves.